TOWARDS QUALITY CARE

Related Titles
in Association with PSSRU

Series Editors:

Professor Martin Knapp, LSE, Professor David Challis, University of
Manchester, Dr Ann Netten, University of Kent

Care Management in Social and Primary Health Care
The Gateshead Community Care Scheme
David Challis, John Chesterman, Rosemary Luckett, Karen Stewart
and Rosemary Chessum
ISBN 1 85742 206 6

Equity and Efficiency Policy in Community Care
Needs, Service Productivities, Efficiencies and Their Implications
Bleddyn Davies and José Fernández
ISBN 0 7546 1281 3

Caring for Older People
An Assessment of Community Care in the 1990s
Linda Bauld, John Chesterman, Bleddyn Davies,
Ken Judge and Roshni Mangalore
ISBN 0 7546 1280 5

Community Care, Secondary Health Care and
Care Management
David Challis, Robin Darton and Karen Stewart
ISBN 1 84014 581 1

This work was undertaken by the PSSRU, which receives support from the
Department of Health; the views expressed in this publication are those of the
authors and not necessarily those of the Department of Health.

Towards Quality Care
Outcomes for Older People in Care Homes

CAROLINE MOZLEY
York Hospitals NHS Trust, UK
formerly PSSRU, University of Manchester, UK

CAROLINE SUTCLIFFE
PSSRU, University of Manchester, UK

HEATHER BAGLEY
PSSRU, University of Manchester, UK

LIS CORDINGLEY
University of Manchester, UK
formerly PSSRU, University of Manchester, UK

DAVID CHALLIS
PSSRU, University of Manchester, UK

PETER HUXLEY
Institute of Psychiatry, UK
formerly PSSRU, University of Manchester, UK

ALISTAIR BURNS
PSSRU, University of Manchester, UK

ASHGATE

Caroline Mozley, Caroline Sutcliffe, Heather Bagley, Lis Cordingley, David Challis, Peter Huxley and Alistair Burns have asserted their right under the Copyright, Designs and Patents Act, 1988, to be identified as the authors of this work.

Published by
Ashgate Publishing Limited
Gower House
Croft Road
Aldershot
Hants GU11 3HR
England

Ashgate Publishing Company
Suite 420
101 Cherry Street
Burlington, VT 05401-4405
USA

Ashgate website: http://www.ashgate.com

British Library Cataloguing in Publication Data
Towards quality care : outcomes for older people in care
   homes
   1. Old age homes - Great Britain - Evaluation 2. Aged - Care
   - Great Britain 3. Aged - Psychology 4. Quality of life
   I. Mozley, Caroline II. University of Kent at Canterbury.
   Personal Social Services Research Unit
   362.6'1'0941

Library of Congress Cataloging-in-Publication Data
Towards quality care : outcomes for older people in care homes / Caroline Mozley ... [et al.].
      p. cm.
   Includes bibliographical references and index.
   ISBN 0-7546-3172-9
      1. Aged–Long-term care–Quality control–Great Britain. 2. Long-term care
   facilities–Quality control–Great Britain. 3. Long-term care of the sick–Quality
   control–Great Britain. 4. Nursing homes–Quality control–Great Britain. 5. Quality
   assurance. I. Mozley, Caroline.

RA998.G7T695 2004
362.16'0941–dc22   2004043703

ISBN 0 7546 3172 9

Typeset by Nick Brawn at the PSSRU, University of Kent
Printed and bound in Great Britain by MPG Books Ltd, Bodmin, Cornwall

Contents

List of Boxes, Figures and Tables

Tables

Foreword

by Elaine Murphy, Chairman, East London and the City Health Authority and Visiting Professor, St Bartholomew's and the Royal London Hospitals Medical and Dental School, Queen Mary.

What makes a good home? Every year in the UK, some thousands of older people, the vast majority with a degree of mental impairment as a result of dementia, leave their own homes for good to go into a residential care home or nursing home. The decision is rarely made solely by the individual and in many cases it is essentially the choice of close relatives or health and social services professional staff. The authors report here an important government funded study designed to throw light on the vexed and complex question of what characteristics determine whether a home provides good quality of care and explore the characteristics of that even more elusive nirvana, homes in which the residents experience an enriching and enjoyable life in their final months and years in spite of profound disabilities.

The research team's findings are satisfyingly clear and direct, and reassuringly make intuitive good sense. At the risk of over-simplification, the research team found that the key quality of a home where residents are happy to contemplate staying for a long time and where staff felt part of a highly cohesive team and enjoyed working is characterised by having a lot of things for residents to do. Daily occupation and opportunities for social interaction are crucial elements which make the difference, a difference which is important enough to influence mortality and whether they become depressed or not. This holds good even when levels of dependency have been taken into account. In other words, having something to do is a life or death matter.

In this study, it was not the physical environment, not the number or qualifications of the staff, not the ethos or specific care practices but opportunities for pleasurable activities. And doesn't this make good common sense? These are homes where there is a satisfying bustle, where staff are engaged in conversation and daily mutual banter with residents, where even the most disabled person is brought into an exercise or music group and included in outings, where the televisions are kept out of sight in residents' private rooms. These are homes where relatives are in and out and welcome and time flies by for both residents and staff, who are busily stretched, tired at the shift's end, but know they are doing a rewarding and worthwhile if tough job. Most professionals in the field have visited homes like this, rare though they are, but are all too familiar with the converse, homes 'like a morgue', a slang expression which takes on new meaning once the implications of this study have been understood.

The recommendations of this study are few and the main one, that homes should be required to provide staff whose sole responsibility is to provide activities and entertainment for residents, will be unpopular in some quarters because it requires resources. The data here are too convincing to allow a criticism of 'unaffordable' to lie unchallenged. Many homes are run too cheaply to provide more than the bare minimum of supervision. Local authorities must take seriously the cost of such services in their contracts and in their criteria for registering a home. Quality care may not require huge investment but it cannot be provided on the cheap.

The report's other recommendations are familiar but important and necessary pleas, first for the universal recognition that all residential and nursing homes provide a service predominantly for people with mental disorder, whether specially designated for elderly people with mental illness or not. Ninety per cent of residents in this study sample had cognitive impairment and nearly a quarter were both demented and depressed. That has been true now for a quarter of a century and it seems astonishing that nursing staff can 'qualify' without formal study of the common psychiatric disorders of late life and only a small fraction of nursing and care assistants receive training in the management of these disorders.

Older residents who pay for their own care are rather less likely to be highly dependent on admission to care. People who might well be judged by health and social services professionals to be capable of independent living if provided with the right combination of daily domestic and personal help at home, are still going into residential care. Is this because, having assessed the alternative options, individuals are making a real choice of communal life for the reassurance of round-the-clock staff or is it as we might suspect, a matter of decisions being made in ignorance of the possibilities of remaining in ones' own home? The authors suggest that all those proposing to enter residential care should have a comprehensive assessment before the decision is irrevocable. This is all well and good but who is going to ensure that this happens in the independent sector where statutory sector professionals are not involved in the decision to enter care? The single assessment process may address these questions. As always, a thoughtful piece of research raises important policy issues to which local authorities and the health service need to give further thought.

The research at PSSRU is noted for its methodological rigour, in a field where there is no shortage of poorly constructed and statistically dubious research published, and the authors should be congratulated on producing such a compelling and readable report. It is a privilege to introduce this careful and painstaking study which is unique in its focus and scale and which should transform the ethos and culture of long-term institutional care for older people.

Acknowledgements

A research project of this size cannot be achieved without the help and co-operation of a large number of people and organisations. First in the list must come the residential and nursing homes in which the study was carried out. For the kindness and patience shown by all the owners, managers, staff and residents, members of the research team are extremely grateful.

Several organisations, including local authorities and private and voluntary sector care providers in the South Manchester, South Cheshire and Blackpool, Wyre and Fylde areas were generous in allowing access to their homes and in supporting the project generally.

The Advisory Group was invaluable in guiding the project throughout. Thanks are due to its members, Professor Mary Marshall, Mr Tony James, Professor Jenny Firth-Cozens, Dr Ann Netten, Mr Robin Darton and Ms Sarah Holme.

For their invaluable help in pilot-testing, our gratitude is owed to the staff and residents of the Alexian Brothers Home in Manchester.

Dr Leonie Price carried out the Geriatric Mental State Schedule interviewing and classified and coded all the diagnosis and medication data.

Statistical advice was provided by Professor Graham Dunn, Dr Brian Farragher and Mr Hadi Mohammed.

Mr Hadi Mohammed provided computer and data management support.

Ms Sherrill Evans coded the returned staff questionnaires.

Dr Siobhan Reilly assisted with the pilot-testing.

Professor Alan Bryman, Loughborough University, advised on leadership research and the interviewing of home managers.

Dr Carol Borill and the staff of the NHS Workforce Survey team at the Institute of Occupational Psychology, University of Sheffield, provided assistance with the construction of the Staff Questionnaire.

Dr Ashley Weinberg's helpful suggestions contributed to the analysis of the data in Chapter 6.

Ms Rebekah Proctor, Dr Jane Byrne and Dr Greta Rait provided training in use of the Geriatric Mental State Schedule.

Kwik Save Stores Ltd generously provided £1,000 in store vouchers to use as draw prizes for staff completing the Staff Questionnaire.

Mrs Pat Mellor, Hearing Therapist at Withington Hospital, Manchester provided advice and amplification equipment which made it possible for some very deaf older people to be interviewed.

The project could not have been carried out without the outstanding diligence and administrative expertise (not to mention good humour) of our project secretary, Mrs Gill Dunkerley, to whom our very particular thanks must go.

Parts of some of the chapters have previously been published as journal articles. We are grateful to the following publishers for permission to reprint all or part of the articles here, with appropriate contextual alterations:

(1) Carfax Publishing Company for permission substantially to reproduce in Chapter 5 the article 'Psychiatric symptomatology in elderly people admitted to nursing and residential homes', first published in *Ageing and Mental Health*, 4, 2, 136–141.

(2) Oxford University Press for permission substantially to reproduce in Chapter 5 the article 'Dependency in older people recently admitted to care homes', first published in *Age and Ageing*, 29, 255–260.

(3) John Wiley and Sons Limited for permission substantially to reproduce in Chapter 9 the article '"Not knowing where I am doesn't mean I don't know what I like": cognitive impairment and quality of life responses in elderly people', first published in *The International Journal of Geriatric Psychiatry*, 14, 776–783.

(4) Blackwell Science Limited for permission substantially to reproduce in pages 139 to 144 the article 'Recognition of depression by staff in nursing and residential homes', first published in *The Journal of Clinical Nursing*, 9, 445–450.

(5) Springer Publishing Company for permission substantially to reproduce in pages 144 to 149 the article 'A new version of the Geriatric Depression Scale for nursing and residential home populations: the Geriatric Depression Scale (Residential) (GDS-12R)', first published in *International Psychogeriatrics*, 2, 173–181.

The project was funded under the National Health Service Executive National Mental Health Programme.

Caroline Mozley, Caroline Sutcliffe, Heather Bagley,
Lis Cordingley, David Challis, Peter Huxley and Alistair Burns

Postscript

This was a challenging project which demanded a high level of commitment from the project research team. In particular the core team — Caroline Mozley, Caroline Sutcliffe, Heather Bagley and Lis Cordingley — made this study possible with their enthusiasm, organisation and high standards. In addition, all the project team would wish to acknowledge the unique contribution made by Caroline Mozley who was a driving force and inspiration from the inception to the completion of the study. A crucial contribution was made by Caroline Sutcliffe who has taken the key responsibility of the final drafting of this manuscript with an exceptional degree of care, diligence and unfailing good humour. This book is a reflection of their contribution.

The manuscript was typeset by Nick Brawn at the PSSRU with his usual skill.

Professor David Challis

1 Quality in Care Homes for Older People

For many years researchers have tried, with varying degrees of success, to throw light on the question of what constitutes good quality long-term care for older people. Much is known about the nature of life in care and those who live in it. However the vast majority of studies in this field have been cross-sectional in design — based on the collection of data on one occasion. The data collection has often been extremely detailed and painstaking, involving interviews of all or a sample of residents, interviews of staff, or direct observation of facilities, residents and staff. Cross-sectional work is designed to provide detailed description and comparison between facilities. It does not look at the outcome of care, the changes and effects experienced by residents arising from the care they receive.

To study care quality issues by means of cross-sectional research design requires the making of *a priori* judgements about what is, or is not, good quality. Care environments can then be described, using various measurement techniques, in terms of the extent to which they do, or do not match up to these predetermined criteria. However there are some problems with this approach. While there is a substantial body of research that supports the view that certain aspects of care are good — provision of privacy being only one example — there is less understanding about the relative importance of, and relationship between, these characteristics. Is privacy more important than good food?... than a good response to physical health needs?... than provision of occupation and activity opportunities? Clearly these are not mutually exclusive and most people would hope that a good quality home pays attention to all these aspects, but are some key areas more important than others? — where quality enhancement efforts should be concentrated because they have a cumulative

1

effect and impact upon quality more generally? A variety of sources can address these questions.

The history of institutional care for older people in the UK is such that much relevant material is to be found in reports of hospital based studies, as well as in work carried out in residential and nursing homes. Some research which has concerned care of children or of people with learning disabilities is also relevant. The disciplinary range is wide, necessitating coverage of medical, social, nursing and psychological research, and the search is by no means confined to UK sources. No attempt will therefore be made in this book to provide a comprehensive review of the literature on residential care of older people. The UK literature has been well reviewed by others, for example Goldberg and Connelly (1982), Sinclair (1990) and Peace et al. (1997). The focus of this book is upon the different ways in which care homes may improve quality of life for older residents.

The definition and measurement of quality in institutional care

One of the earliest attempts to produce a global assessment or 'score' of institutional quality is to be found in *The Last Refuge* (Townsend, 1962). This was based on a comprehensive survey of local authority residential accommodation for older people in the late 1950s, for which visits were made to a representative sample of 173 homes in England and Wales. The research team's interviews with residents, staff and managers and their observation of facilities and regimes produced a wealth of descriptive material which makes the book an invaluable historical document. For present purposes, however, what is of interest is the Provisional Measure of an Institution's Quality. Taking into account a large number of physical and organisational variables, quality scores were awarded to each home out of a possible maximum of 100, with a score of 60 or more indicating an acceptable standard. This was one of the first attempts to do this sort of thing and Townsend acknowledged both the complexity of the undertaking and the shortcomings of the measure. He pointed out that while it is possible to standardise a method for collecting comparable data on a wide range of variables it is another matter to attach weightings to them so as to produce a quality measure. More than 40 years later this problem remains.

There have been many subsequent attempts to measure quality, some of them comprehensive measures or measurement packages and others concentrating on specific aspects of institutional life. The more global measures include Linn's (1966, 1977) Nursing Home Rating Scale; Booth's (1985) Institutional Regimes Questionnaire and the Quality Measurement Schedule used by Willcocks et al. (1987). A more limited approach to global measurement is exemplified by Challiner et al. (1994) who used an 18-item quality evaluation schedule for a postal questionnaire. Working in the field of services for people with learning disabilities, Wolfensberger and his colleagues (1972, 1978) developed the concept of 'normalisation' as the goal of institutional provision. Their Programme Analysis of Service Systems was designed for quantitative evaluation of services in terms of their promotion of normalisation.

Perhaps the most comprehensive package of assessment instruments is the Multiphasic Environmental Assessment Procedure (Moos, 1974; Moos et al., 1979; Moos and Lemke, 1992), refined over a number of years at Stanford University. Based on a social ecology perspective, this provides a method for systematic collection of data for use in evaluating residential institutions. It does require slight modification for use in a non-American context but a number of UK researchers, including Benjamin and Spector (1990) and Netten (1993), have found that aspects of the package, particularly the Sheltered Care Environment Scale, transfer with few cultural or linguistic problems. This instrument is central to evaluation of the 'social climate' of homes, a process for which Timko and Moos (1991a, b) offered a six-category classification system, characterising homes as 'supportive, self-directed', 'supportive, well organised', 'open conflict', 'suppressed conflict', 'emergent positive' or 'unresponsive'.

A number of researchers have taken a less global approach to the study of institutional quality. Social interaction has been studied by means of interview (for example, Henderson et al., 1981) and a number of different observation methods (Godlove et al., 1982; Clark and Bowling, 1990; Dean et al., 1993) which have also investigated the activities of staff and residents.

Some quality measures have been developed with the express intention of facilitating audit activity or quality enhancement training programmes. These do not always lend themselves to use in a more 'arm's length' research context. In the *Co-operative Quality Assurance Study* for long-term care (Chambers, 1984, 1986) direct care providers took a total of 4.5 hours using the procedure to review their standards for one health problem treated as a proxy for quality, obtained information about compliance with the standard for seven residents, and finished with group discussion. *Evaluating the Quality of Care: A Self Assessment Manual* (Payne et al., 1994) is similarly designed as a tool for use by care providers. Based on work done as part of the *Caring in Homes Initiative* (Youll and McCourt-Perring, 1993), it offers a comprehensive programme for assessing all aspects of a home's operation.

Instruments that can be used to evaluate aspects of the care in a home are to be found in the literature on nursing and medical audit procedures, an area that has expanded greatly during the last decade. A number of relevant instruments arising from the speciality of psychiatric nursing are reviewed by Balogh et al. (1993). The Royal College of Physicians and the British Geriatrics Society (1992) in their jointly produced guidelines and audit measures for long-term care took the approach of specifying eight key indicators of quality care which are largely, but not exclusively, health-related. The specific guidelines for practice in each of these areas are designed to be audited using the

Continuous Assessment, Review and Evaluation audit package (Hopkins et al., 1992).

Regulation and approaches to quality

The provision of high quality care in residential and nursing homes and the regulation and maintenance of standards in them is a source of concern for societies around the globe. Quality indicators may be seen in terms of Donabedian's (1980) criteria of structure, process and outcome. In the UK, early quality measures were concerned purely with structure, factors such as allocation of space and fire regulations. The introduction of a code of practice for residential care, _Home Life_ (Centre for Policy on Ageing, 1984), following the Registered Homes Act 1984, formally introduced more process-based measures providing standards for physical and social care, with a focus on the dignity of the residents. This was further developed in an independent review of care homes (Wagner, 1988). Both of these influenced the inspection model _Homes Are For Living In_ (Department of Health/SSI, 1989) which shaped the content of the inspection process employed until 2002. This was extended with the publication of the consultation document _Fit for the Future_ (Department of Health, 1999) on national standards for residential and nursing homes. Further standards were developed following the policy commitment to greater consistency and clarity in care across England (Cm 4169, 1998) with national minimum care standards. These were established following the Care Standards Act (2000) containing structural measures such as 'environment' and 'staffing', and process measures such as 'health and personal care', and 'daily life and social activities'. These standards are arranged under seven key topics: Choice of Home; Health and Personal Care; Daily Life and Social Activities; Complaints and Protection; Environment; Staffing; and Management and Administration (Department of Health, 2001a). Overall this produces 38 standards. Of these indicators, the nine standards arranged under 'Health and Personal Care' and 'Daily Life and Social Activities' approximate most closely to the traditional resident-centred definition of quality of life. They cover: the existence of a care plan; health care; medication; privacy and dignity; dying and death; social contact and activities; community contact; autonomy and choice; meals and mealtimes. Each standard has a broad outcome statement with more precise indications of how this is operationalised. The strategy is designed to shift towards standards that 'focus on the key areas that most affect the quality of life experienced by service users, as well as physical standards' (Cm 4169, 1998, para 4.48).

In other countries similar approaches have been employed. For example, in Israel a tracer approach is adopted to identify quality problems in four key areas: nursing/medical; psycho-social; environmental/operational; and organisational (Fleishman et al., 1995). Examples within each domain respectively include mobility and incontinence; loneliness and degree of resident involvement; food and laundry; and furnishings and recording systems. However, individual resident information is only collected on a sample basis and therefore does not link the regulatory requirements with resident quality of life.

In the US, incentives have been provided to nursing homes through additional reimbursement to make quality improvements beyond certain minimum standards. However, such approaches suffer from a focus at the institutional rather than the resident level, and also from problems about the reliability and validity of the indicators used to measure quality (Geron, 1991). Attempts have also been made to link reimbursement of homes to quality of care provided on an outcome basis. In practice this can mean offering incentives for the pursuit of care goals presumed to be associated with good resident outcomes (a process based approach to quality), or for the achievement of outcomes for individual residents which are higher than would otherwise have been expected (an outcome based approach) (Kane et al., 1983; Kane and Kane, 1987). In practice it appears that the administration costs of such an approach are high and that there are difficulties in achieving sufficiently robust outcome indicators (Kane and Kane, 1988).

Also in the US, a more resident focused approach has been employed using the Minimum Data Set/Resident Assessment Instrument (MDS/RAI) (Morris et al., 1990). The instrument is used in US Nursing Homes for residents on entry and again at regular intervals. The MDS consists of 20 domains of assessment of need which may trigger more detailed assessment of need using assessment protocols. A UK version is available (Challis et al., 2000a). The assessment information is used to develop individual care plans and at an aggregated level as part of the quality assurance process by US state governments. Thus, routine regulatory information is supplemented by quality indicators derived from individual resident assessment information (Zimmerman et al., 1995; Karon and Zimmerman, 1996), covering care domains such as psychotropic drug use and physical functioning.

The Quality of Life Study

In the absence of an external 'gold standard' or touchstone by which quality is judged these issues come down to matters of judgement by and consensus of researchers and professionals. Not only is this intuitively inadequate but there is some evidence that expert judges have a poor record for consistency in rating quality home care (Gibbs and Sinclair, 1992a, b). The Quality of Life Study was based on the premiss that the only way to make proper judgements of quality is by looking at outcomes. Rather than making *a priori* judgements about factors which do or do not constitute quality care or about where quality care is to be found, this study set out to investigate the effects of care on its recipients. Good quality care was defined, not as care that provides privacy and independence, not care in homes with a high staff ratio — but care which produces a good outcome.

Intuitively, the criteria identifying a good outcome of care suggest themselves without much difficulty. Residents should be maintained in the best possible:

- physical functioning;
- mental health;
- cognitive functioning; and
- quality of life.

In addition, with long-term care increasingly accessed and paid for directly by residents and their relatives rather than through professional intermediaries it was decided to investigate a secondary outcome — production of high levels of confidence and satisfaction in residents' relatives.

The original design of the study was influenced by the Production of Welfare (PoW) framework in relation to residential and nursing home care. In essence, the PoW approach argues that outcomes (in this case Quality of Life) are determined by the combination of resource inputs (such as staff, the physical qualities of the building and other capital), and non resource inputs (such as the management style, activities and social environment of the home) (Davies and Knapp, 1980; Challis et al., 1988; Challis and Darton, 1990). The approach is helpful in framing a causal relationship between the aspects of resource inputs, non resource inputs, quality of care and quality of life.

By investigating change over time in a large cohort of residents following admission to a variety of nursing and residential homes, the study set out to determine whether achievement of the desired outcomes was more likely in some care environments than in others — and to identify the particular characteristics of care most likely to be associated with best outcome.

The task of investigating differences in resident outcomes involved a two-phase programme of interviews — the baseline and the follow up. During the 15-month baseline period all residents newly admitted to the studied homes were referred to the project so that they could be interviewed within 14 days. Follow-up interviews were done five and nine months after admission. The interviews and associated data collected during the baseline assessment formed the basis of a cross-sectional study of new admissions; the follow-up data were used for the longitudinal, or outcome analysis.

The relevance of the study

The study is particularly relevant in the light of the quality agenda which has become part of the government's Modernisation Strategy in Health and Social Care in England (Cm 4169, 1998). Quality of care and quality of life are perennial areas of concern given particular emphasis at present in the light of the focus upon quality in government policy over recent years. Quality has been a key tenet of the government's modernisation programme and has been evident in a number of fields such as the NHS (Department of Health, 1998a), and the introduction of the *Quality Protects* programme in services for vulnerable children (Department of Health, 1998b). The introduction of the Best Value approach established upon local councils a duty to deliver services by the most effective, economic and efficient approach taking into account quality and cost. It is intended to emphasise continuous improvement (Cm 4014, 1998). The White Paper *Modernising Social Services* (Cm 4169, 1998) identified a number of themes related to quality including a focus on: services that promote independence and are consistent and fit individual needs; improvement in regulation and inspection; and the improvement of standards in the workforce. The 'Quality Strategy' developed by the UK government in the field of social care (Department of Health, 2000) builds upon the latter White Paper. It focuses upon the three themes of enhancing the consistency of social services, creating more accessible and individually tailored services, and enhancing the skills and competencies of the workforce. The quality agenda is to be supported by the National Care Standards Commission, promoting minimum standards; the Social Care Institute of Excellence (SCIE), collating knowledge and developing guidelines; the General Social Care Council (GSCC) developing codes of conduct and regulating social work training; and the National Training Organisation for Personal Social Services (TOPSS), responsible for producing occupational standards.

The current focus on quality is underpinned with a concern for 'what works', defined in terms of services which produce valued outcomes for those who use them and for their carers. The Quality of Life Study was designed to provide evidence on effective practice in care homes that leads to better outcomes in terms of quality of life of those older people who use those services.

The structure of this book

Chapter 2 discusses the issues involved in studying quality of life of older people and the outcomes of residential care. In Chapter 3 the design and methods used in the study are described. Chapters 4 and 5 make use of the baseline data to describe the homes and their residents. The data analysed and presented here stand in their own right as a detailed cross-sectional picture of a large cohort of newly admitted residents and of the care which they received. In addition, these chapters explain the derivation of the variables used for the subsequent longitudinal analysis which was the main purpose of the study. The staff questionnaire, completed by 440 staff about half-way through the 15 month baseline period provides the basis of Chapters 6 and 7; Chapter 8 reports the views of residents' relatives.

Chapters 9 and 10 describe some specific analyses carried out using the baseline data, concerning the relationship between cognitive impairment and 'interviewability' on quality of life subjects, the response of staff to depressive symptoms, and the development of an effective measure of depression in care homes. Chapter 11 deals with the longitudinal analysis which links outcomes to the characteristics of the home and the individual residents. Multivariate techniques are used to investigate relationships between resident outcomes and the characteristics of the care environment, broadly defined. Chapter 12 considers the findings of the study in the light of current developments in the long-term care of older people.

2 Quality of Life in Residential and Nursing Home Care

The last few years have seen a proliferation of interest in quality of life research, particularly in relation to provision of medical and care services. This interest has not been confined to researchers and professionals but has engaged the media and general public. This chapter examines aspects of health and dependency of older people, quality of life research generally, and some recent studies of quality of life in residential and nursing homes.

The dependency, psychiatric and physical needs of elderly people in institutional care

Dependency

Numerous studies have demonstrated a gradient of dependency for vulnerable older people between care settings such as home care, residential homes, nursing homes and hospital wards (Charlesworth and Wilkin, 1982; Bond et al., 1989; Stott et al., 1990; Philp et al., 1991; Campbell Stern et al., 1993). Most recently, studies have suggested that there is an increase in dependency in residents admitted to residential and nursing homes from the mid-1980s to the late 1990s (Netten et al., 2001a). Although there is a considerable overlap in the dependency of residents in residential and nursing homes, older people entering nursing homes are on average more dependent than those entering residential homes (Netten et al., 2001b). These dependency attributes are reflected in the physical and psychiatric morbidity which has been identified in the residents of care homes.

As might be expected, there is a higher prevalence of disease in older people than in any other age group and the situation is further complicated by the presence of multiple pathology, increased severity, co-morbidity of mental and physical illness and iatrogenic disorders. Although mortality rates at older ages have fallen (Frischer, 1991) the extra years are often accompanied by illness and disability.

Psychiatric disorders

The most common psychiatric illnesses encountered in older people are delirium, dementia and depression. These are not mutually exclusive and often co-exist.

Delirium is an acquired, global impairment of memory, intellect and personality with impaired consciousness, the cause invariably being physical. The onset of delirium is acute, distinguishing it from dementia in which onset is gradual (Baldwin, 1997). The most frequent precipitants are pneumonia, congestive cardiac failure, urinary tract infection, dietary factors and carcinomatosis. The main predictive factors are dementia, defective hearing and vision and Parkinson's disease. Mortality is high (Henderson, 1986).

Dementia describes a clinical syndrome characterised by problems with memory and other intellectual functions, psychiatric symptoms and behavioural disturbances, and difficulties in activities of daily living. There are three main causes — Alzheimer's disease, vascular dementia and Lewy Body dementia. Other rarer causes include Huntington's disease, Creutzfeldt-Jacob Disease, Pick's disease and dementia associated with Parkinson's disease.

Dementia may be regarded as a terminal illness, with research indicating differing mortality rates according to such factors as type of dementia and age at onset (Burns and Lewis, 1993). A study of new referrals to a psychogeriatric service, carried out over 15 years, found mortality rates for Alzheimer's disease ranged between 53, 81, 98 and 100 per cent, at 2, 5, 10 and 15 years respectively (Robinson, 1989). Eagles et al. (1990), in a case-control study of cognitive impairment in people over 65 years, found that those with cognitive impairment were 3.5 times more likely to die than those without cognitive impairment, although there was not a specific association between dementia and increased mortality. It has been shown that people with Alzheimer's disease have less physical illness than those with affective disorders, but that those with vascular dementia have more (Roth and Kay, 1956). The commonest cause of death in Alzheimer's disease is pneumonia (Burns et al., 1990). In one survey of psychiatric illness in residential homes in London (Mann et al., 1984) one-third of residents had severe dementia, one-third mild to moderate dementia and only one-third were cognitively intact. Of the latter two-thirds, 38 per cent were depressed. The prevalence rate of dementia increased with age and was higher among women.

Depression, according to the generally accepted diagnostic criteria embodied in ICD [International Classification of Diseases] 10, is a collection of symptoms affecting mood, appetite, weight, energy, concentration and cognition. It is relatively common in later life (Gelder et al., 1989), when its symptomatology is characterised by more agitation and hypochondriasis. Depression affects around five per cent of the population aged over 65, with 2–3 per cent being severely affected, but reaches much higher proportions in patients in surgical or medical wards and also in residential and nursing homes (Baldwin, 1997). First depressive illness is less common after the age of 60 and rare after the age of 80 (Savartz and Blazer, 1986). It is more common in older women than in older men (Freedman et al., 1982), continuing the gender difference pattern seen in younger age groups (Paykel, 1991). Chronic physical illness, impaired vision and hearing loss are all major aetiological factors (Roth and Kay, 1956).

Among residents of residential homes, Mann et al. (1984) found that depression was more common in residents admitted from their own homes or belonging to a minority religion. Residents who had been in a home for the longest period were least affected by depression, perhaps suggesting recovery from depression after a period of adjustment, or that depression too is predictive of shorter life expectancy in older age. This and other studies (Schneider et al., 1997a, b, c; Mann et al., 2000) suggest that many depressive disorders go undetected or are regarded as part of normal ageing and that, as a result, depression remains under-treated in residential homes. Evidence from the US suggests that the mental health of very old people is particularly neglected (Burns and Lewis, 1993). Depressive illness in older people, if treated adequately, responds very well, with up to 85 per cent showing considerable improvement after treatment (Murphy, 1983). A good prognosis is associated with age below 70, short duration of illness and absence of physical illness. Poor prognosis is associated with a severe episode of depression and poor physical health. Improvements to the nursing home environment in terms of greater resident choice and independent decision-making, and better education, training and retention of qualified nursing staff, have been suggested as ways to address incidence of late-onset depression in nursing home residents (Bell and Goss, 2001).

Physical disorders

There are many physical illnesses, acute and chronic, that are common in old age. The commonest cause of death in older people is cardiovascular disease (for example myocardial infarction, cerebrovascular accident, cardiac failure), followed by malignant neoplasms (Thomas et al., 1986). Other common conditions include osteoarthritis, visual and auditory impairment, incontinence, diabetes, Parkinson's disease and infections (for example pneumonia, urinary tract infection and infective gastro-intestinal disease.) Around 25 per cent of long-term care residents are hospitalised at least once in the second six months of their stay, the primary diagnoses being cardiac failure and respiratory disease (Fried and Mor, 1997).

Many chronic physical illnesses have a profound effect on mobility and thus on the general quality of life of elderly people. Reduced mobility also increases risk of falling. One in four people over 65 in the community fall — those over 75 years in institutions fall more frequently. Many falls are a direct result of acute illness, medication and environmental hazards. Morbidity can be considerable (Ulfarsson and Robinson, 1994).

Infectious disease is also common in residential care settings. For instance, 95 per cent of outbreaks of infectious gastro-intestinal disease in residential settings occur in homes for older people (Ryan et al., 1997). Influenza epidemics are associated with excess winter mortality and both chronic illness and living in residential care are associated risk factors. Influenza vaccination of high-risk groups has been shown to decrease mortality by 41 per cent overall and up to 75 per cent in those previously vaccinated (Ahmed et al., 1995). Thus an adequate vaccination programme can do much to reduce mortality in older people.

The relationship between co-morbidity and survival of American nursing home patients with dementia was studied over eight years by Van Dijk et al. (1996). The 2-year survival rates for men and women were found to be 60 per cent and 39 per cent respectively. Parkinson's disease, atrial fibrillation, pulmonary infection and malignancy were powerful predictors, more or less doubling mortality. Patients who had suffered a stroke and also had a chest infection had a particularly poor prognosis. Severely demented patients had more co-morbidity than those less severely affected but the impact of co-morbidity on survival did not depend on the severity of dementia. Patients admitted directly from hospital had more co-morbidity and were more severely demented than those coming from home. Co-morbidity and severity of dementia were found independently to influence mortality. In a study of 3-year mortality of over 1000 community residents aged over 65, Dewey et al. (1993) found that 'expressed wish to die' was a predictor of mortality, controlling for age, sex and cognitive impairment. Patients with moderate to severe physical morbidity are at increased risk of developing psychiatric illness and when physical illness is present, psychiatric symptoms are more severe (Murphy, 1983).

Quality of life research

The conceptual background

The Concise Oxford Dictionary defines quality as 'degree of excellence, relative nature or kind or character'. One may talk of high or low quality of life, or compare quality of life between countries or social groups, but there is still much debate about what 'quality of life' actually means. Attempts to measure or define quality of life need to 'take into account the subject's culture, expectations, beliefs, and desires, as well as the many limitations to achieving his or her wishes and state of mind' (Wade, 1992).

A common theme in the attempt to describe quality of life is the interaction between its objective and subjective determinants: '... a person's existential state, well-being, satisfaction with life, or whatever is determined on the one hand by the exogenous (objective) facts and factors of his life, and on the other hand by the endogenous (subjective) perception and assessment he has of these facts and factors of life and of himself' (Szalai, 1980). Furthermore, quality of life, it has been argued, could be 'defined in terms of what one has lost, or lacks, rather than what one has', particularly with regard to comparison with other people (Bowling and Windsor, 2001).

Like many others, Draper (1992) questions what visible aspects of quality of life should be chosen as its indicators and how we can justify this choice, and sees the profusion of quality of life measures as reflecting, 'a fractured perception of human being'. Farquhar (1995a) in her review of definitions of quality of life identifies four main types:

- *Global definitions*, which refer simply to one's overall degree of satisfaction or dissatisfaction with aspects of one's life (Abrams, 1973).
- *Component definitions*, which break quality of life down into its component parts or identify particular characteristics which are thought to be important in the evaluation of quality of life. For example George and Bearon (1980) define quality of life in terms of four dimensions, two of which are objective and two of which reflect personal judgement of the individual.
- *Focused definitions*, which refer particularly to specific components, the commonest types being health and functional ability, often referred to as 'health-related quality of life'.
- *Combination definitions*, which do not fit into any of the above categories or overlap more than one definition.

Within quality of life literature, there is not only debate about what the concept means, but multiplicity of terminology, with references made to 'life satisfaction', and 'well-being' among other terms. The main terms in common use have been defined in the following ways.

Life satisfaction: A number of studies have used life satisfaction as a measure of life quality (Andrews and Withey, 1976). Neugarten (1974) viewed life satisfaction for older people as the extent to which they took pleasure from activities that constitute daily life, regarded life as meaningful, felt they had succeeded in achieving major life goals, held positive self-image and regard, and maintained an optimistic attitude. Cantril (1965) defined life satisfaction as the extent to which people's perceptions of their current lives coincide with their definitions of the best possible life, and developed 'Cantril's ladder' as a uni-dimensional measure of this. George and Bearon (1980) saw life satisfaction as one dimension of quality of life. They regarded life satisfaction, morale, and happiness as global concepts referring to life as a whole rather than specific domains of life experience which, because of their global nature, may be of limited use in evaluative research. For example if life satisfaction and morale are relatively stable personality traits rather than 'reactive and manipulable' they will be unaffected by intervention and should not be used for programme evaluation.

Well-being: This has been measured by three major scales; the Life Satisfaction Index (Neugarten et al., 1961), the Bradburn Affect-Balance Scales (Bradburn, 1969) and the Philadelphia Geriatric Center Morale Scale (Lawton, 1975). Bradburn has described his scale as an indicator of happiness or general psychological well-being that is not concerned with detecting psychiatric or psychological disorders.

Happiness: This has been defined as a transitory mood of 'gaiety and elation' that reflects the affect that people feel towards their current state of affairs (Campbell et al., 1976). Happiness implies an affective mood or state, with a more emotional component than a cognitive component (Andrews and McKennel, 1980). Older people often report lower levels of happiness but higher levels of life satisfaction than younger people (Campbell, 1981).

Self-esteem: Self-esteem, according to George and Bearon (1980), is another global concept like life satisfaction, which is one dimension of quality of life. In their view, whether self-esteem is a relatively stable attribute, resistant to changes in one's environment, or a more transient state, has not yet been resolved.

Morale: This has been defined as 'the presence or absence of satisfaction, optimism and expanding life perspectives' by Kutner et al. (1956). Lawton (1975) developed a widely used morale measure and described high morale as 'a basic sense of satisfaction with oneself — a feeling that there is a place in the environment for oneself — that people and things in one's life offer some satisfaction to the individual'.

Approaches to measurement

Approaches to the measurement of quality of life fall into two main categories. The 'profile' approach attempts to measure life quality in different areas or 'domains'. Single measure approaches, often using visual analogue scales of various kinds, are global measures which require subjects to take a single, broad view of how they see their lives. Examples of the first approach are to be found in Bowling (1995) and Oliver et al. (1996).

Several widely used measures of the second type are based on the Rosser Index of Disability and Distress (Rosser and Kind, 1978). Originally an indicator of hospital performance, this was designed as a tool for comparing outcome of health care procedures in a single index over time and gave rise to the concept of the QALY or Quality Adjusted Life Year. For the most part these measures have concentrated on health related quality of life. Spitzer's Quality of Life Index or Uniscale (Spitzer et al., 1981) was designed to fill a gap in available quality of life instruments for use with the seriously ill and has been used in cancer research. It is unsuitable for use with healthy people and its reliability and validity have been questioned (Slevin et al., 1988; Bowling, 1997). The Euroqol (Euroqol Group, 1990) was developed by a transnational multidisciplinary team as a generic (i.e. non-disease specific) measure for use in health care evaluation research. A number of other widely used health related quality of life measures were used in the development of the Euroqol, including the Quality of Well-being Scale (Patrick et al., 1973), the Sickness Impact Profile (Bergner et al., 1976), the Nottingham Health Profile (Hunt et al., 1980, 1986) and the Rosser Index (Rosser and Kind, 1978).

A recent study of the use of the Euroqol with elderly acute care patients was carried out to assess ability to self-complete, construct validity and sensitivity to change (Coast et al., 1998). With regard to construct validity, the Euroqol was found to be highly correlated with the Barthel Activities of Daily Living Index. Most importantly however, the probability of requiring interviewer administration rose in relation to the patient's age, and among those with lower cognitive ability. The authors conclude that if the Euroqol is designed for the measurement of outcome across a range of treatments and diseases, it should be made applicable to all groups of patients, particularly if it is to be used for the development of QALYs.

Single or generic measures have received some criticism from those who believe that quality of life is essentially multi-dimensional and maintain that components of a questionnaire should not be aggregated and summed since each area is measuring a separate construct (Bowling, 1995). Looking at the matter from the perspective of a healthy, rather than a sick, population a national survey on quality of life was carried out with a random sample of 2000 adults. Quality of life was defined as 'the social, psychological and physical domains of life, incorporating a subjective assessment of important life domains in relation to achieving satisfaction'. It included the things that people regarded as important in their lives, both good and bad. The most important things mentioned in response to an open-ended question were respectively; relationships with family and relatives, their own health, the health of a close person, followed by finances/standard of living/housing. When specified options were presented to some respondents as a list, there was a change in the priority of these areas (Bowling, 1995). Bowling and Windsor (2001) subsequently reported that the subjective ratings of life in self-nominated areas of importance explained the most variance in overall quality of life ratings. However, the final model still explained only a small amount of the variance, confirming the complex nature of quality of life. They argue that quality of life measurement scales need to be more sensitive to the differing values of various social groups and changes in priorities that occur with increasing age.

Establishing the validity of quality of life measures has been acknowledged to be problematic since no gold standard exists for comparison (Hughes, 1990; Fletcher et al., 1992; Farquhar, 1995a). Critics assert that the subjective view of the person whose life is being assessed cannot be judged against anything else. Evidence put forward for the validity of quality of life measures has often been restricted to comparison with other similar measures.

Specific issues in relation to older people

If there is debate as to what constitutes quality of life in general, there is similar debate about whether quality of life in old age should be regarded as different in some way from quality of life of younger people. Hughes (1990) has proposed that quality of life of older people should be defined in a similar way to that of younger people; although the experience of being old is shared she cautions against the idea that old age is a 'leveller' and that the experience is the same for all. Other studies have found that younger and older people report similar overall health perceptions despite older people having poorer role function, lower energy levels and poorer physical function when objectively assessed (Mangione et al., 1993).

Studies of older people as a group started to appear in the late 1950s and 1960s with reports by Townsend (1957, 1962) and Tunstall (1966). They found that older people had a poor quality of life (measured objectively), with many living in poverty. Around the same time, some American studies with older people led to the development of disengagement theory (Cumming and

Henry, 1961). This theory proposes that ageing is 'an inevitable mutual withdrawal' or disengagement resulting in decreased interaction between the ageing person and others in the social system he or she belongs to. They studied a sample of 279 healthy Middle Western Americans 'with no economic worries' aged between 50 and 70 and a small sample of 38 people over the age of 80 years. They concluded that their research findings supported the theory of disengagement; elderly people do not replace friends lost through death and as they turn more into themselves, the disengagement process becomes self-perpetuating. Disengagement is different for men and women, and more difficult for men. This theory of old age, which implies that older people should be regarded as a separate group, has been criticised by a number of social gerontologists in recent years (Peace et al.,1979; Clark and Bowling, 1990; Bowling and Formby, 1992).

Most clinical and gerontological researchers differentiate quality of life from purely subjective concepts such as life satisfaction (Gentile, 1991; Patrick and Erickson, 1993; McDowell and Newell, 1996). Frytak (2000) suggests that the definition of quality of life for older people has to be broad and include measures of well-being and of the environment. She suggests that for older people in care home settings more specific formulations are required and cites the work of Kane et al. (1999). They identified 11 outcome domains that would constitute psychosocial quality of life: autonomy/choice; dignity; privacy; individuality; enjoyment; meaningful activity; relationships; sense of sincerity/safety/order; comfort; spiritual well-being; and functional competence. In this work definitions of resident outcome are made explicit and the nursing home processes and practices which are likely to influence each domain are specified. These can be seen to overlap with some of the domains in the UK National Care Standards (Department of Health, 2001a). Frytak (2000) suggests that the work of Lawton (1983, 1991) offers a highly systematic attempt to conceptualise quality of life of older adults. Lawton offers four aspects: behavioural competence; psychological well-being; perceived quality of life; and objective environment. All of these domains were addressed in the Quality of Life Study.

There is also a belief that quality of life in older people can be affected by social class, experience and gender. Living through poverty and deprivation will alter the outlook of some older people compared with those who have lived a more privileged or comfortable life (Hughes, 1990). In a study of a group of older people living at home, Farquhar (1995b) found that quality of life varies according to age group and geographical location. The aim of the study was to gather information about older people's thoughts on quality of life. She asked a sample of people over 65 years to define and describe the quality of their lives in their own words. Forty per cent of the sample described the quality of their lives very positively. The very old tended to describe their lives very negatively compared with the 'younger old'. There were geographical differences, those in semi-rural areas being more positive than those in the inner-city areas. Social contacts and health were given as reasons for having a good quality of life, while ill health or disability were reasons given for having bad quality of life.

A study designed to investigate the multi-dimensional nature of quality of life in very old age was undertaken with a sample of people aged 85 and over living in their own homes in East London. Nine variables which represented three domains of quality of life — 'perceived well-being and autonomy'; 'health and activity', and 'environment' — were selected on the basis of information from focus groups and were measured using well-validated scales. The authors found an association between 'good' quality of life scores and mortality. However, diversity within the relatively homogenous sample of older people confirms the need to take a multi-dimensional perspective on quality of life in old age (Grundy and Bowling, 1999). Other research has supported the view that there is a positive association between perception of health in older people and their quality of life (Moore et al., 1993).

Research has also been undertaken to look specifically at health-related problems of older people in relation to their quality of life. This is an important issue in that it raises the question of whose definition of quality of life in relation to health should be used — the older person's, or the physician's? Pearlman and Uhlmann (1988) looked at quality of life in terms of medical decisions involving a sample of outpatients suffering chronic disease. The patients' ratings of their quality of life were generally higher than physicians' ratings. They suggested that quality of life in older out-patients with chronic diseases is a multi-dimensional construct involving health, as well as social and other factors, and that physicians may misunderstand patients' perceptions of this.

Other researchers have found differences within the medical profession in the assessment of quality of life (Kayser-Jones, 1986). Not only is there little consensus within the medical profession as to what constitutes good quality of life, but also, due to the differences in power between the professional and the patient, it is usually the professional's definition which takes precedence (Clark, 1995). The majority of scales so far have been developed by professionals based upon their definitions and standards, despite the fact that feelings are intrinsic and subjective (Farquhar, 1995b).

The study of quality of life in older people has been described as having the disadvantage of being a 'fashionable concept', with researchers projecting onto it different aspects of meaning (Evans, 1992). The problem arises from the characteristics of older people: questionnaires and interviews designed for use with a general population are more prone to ceiling and floor effects. This is particularly the case with health-related measures which look at functional abilities. In terms of physical disability and dependency, older people may get lower scores which will not change over time, or scores which are unable to discriminate between different levels of disability. There is debate regarding the appropriateness of health-related quality of life measures for older people with regard to instruments that have been designed for a younger population (Bowling, 1998).

In general, some quality of life research has shown that people may not always tell the truth, may be influenced by the question framework, or may give an answer which they think is expected of them (Andrews and Withey, 1976). Older people have a tendency to give optimistic estimates of their state of health and well-being. Although older people may have lower expectations of their lives, this is not a valid reason for not asking them about their quality of life. Furthermore, Evans (1992) queried whether older people should remain in a state with which they report satisfaction despite the belief that the situation could be improved.

Fallowfield (1991) believes that the three major concomitants of old age that profoundly affect quality of life are physical and mental deterioration, retirement and bereavement. Good health probably contributes more to overall quality of life than anything else, yet it is important to consider how much a particular disease or symptom interferes with everyday tasks when measuring the quality of a person's life. For example, developing angina may have a major impact on a previously sporty person, but this is insignificant compared to someone who cannot bend or see to read. Improving quality of life may be as simple as providing suitable aids and appliances. With the correct aids and environment, people with poor mobility may be able to get around very well with little help (Denham, 1991). Retirement from full-time work is a major life event which results in significant changes to a person's life, often involving a change in roles. Not only is there loss associated with retirement, but older people often suffer bereavements of family and friends, which are associated with an increase in illness and mortality (Fallowfield, 1991).

Mental health is also an important consideration in quality of life of older people. The common problems of depression and dementia must be taken into account in any assessment of quality of life, although the direction of causation is often unclear. Arguably both disorders result in lowered quality of life. However the effect can also be seen in the opposite direction — depressed people may tend to view the world in a poor light and report low quality of life as a result of the illness. Similarly, dementia can affect an individual's ability to appraise his situation and this may affect their outlook and responses to quality of life questions (Denham, 1991).

Donaldson et al. (1988) found that the categories of the Rosser Index could not discriminate between older people in long-term care and that scores on the Life Satisfaction Index were unobtainable for almost three-quarters of the sample after nine months due to death and mental frailty. They concluded that measuring quality of life in residential settings is fraught with difficulties including the 'unthinking compliance of respondents' and the fact that the disability state of an older person may remain fairly static over time. Measuring quality of life is further complicated by the fact that different types of long-term care are unlikely to have much effect on life expectancy. Combined with an insensitive measure, this could mean that long-term care of older people scores poorly in terms of QALYs gained when compared to acute care, and this, the authors believe, could lead to discrimination in terms of resource allocation if based on the QALY in its present form.

Thus quality of life may not be appropriate as the sole outcome measure in older people. When Clark and Bowling (1989) carried out a comparative trial of nursing home care versus conventional geriatric ward care, quality of life was shown to be better in the nursing home setting, yet there was also faster functional deterioration. The choice of outcome measures may ultimately depend upon the goals of care, for example quality of life rather than length of survival, and may be influenced by vested interests in the delivery of health care (Evans, 1992).

Some recent quality of life studies in residential care

In spite of the conceptual and methodological challenges, a number of research studies on the quality of life of older people have been carried out in institutional care settings. Some of these studies have excluded older people with mental or physical frailty (for example Philp et al., 1989) whereas others have ensured that all qualify for inclusion (for example Barry et al., 1993). Quality of life has been investigated in relation to the degree to which residents maintain independence and self-respect within the home environment. These factors can be affected by prevalence of dementia and physical dependency among the residents, staff attitudes and the physical structure of the environment. This complicated relationship illustrates the 'complex interaction between the characteristics of the individual and his or her environment' (Fletcher et al., 1992).

Freedom of choice and control have been central themes in a number of studies. In one American study (Cox et al., 1991), a sample of residents in a large nursing home were permanently assigned nursing assistants with a case manager nurse, shifts were altered to accommodate residents' preferences, and staff focused on the needs of residents rather than the procedures involved in their care. Residents in the experimental group reported significant increases in control, choice and well-being unlike those in the comparison group. Post intervention, staff on the experimental unit expressed a more positive attitude towards resident control and choice, and perceived their quality of care to be higher. The authors concluded that the resident's degree of control over a situation is an important factor in a good outcome, and suggested that this model of care could be provided to all residents without additional costs.

However, there is not always agreement between nursing staff and residents on the value placed on freedom of choice and control. Oleson and colleagues (1994) used a semi-structured questionnaire with mentally competent residents, and registered nursing staff. The main question asked was: 'what things are important to a good quality of life for older persons living in institutions?' The most frequently mentioned category by both nurses and residents was 'individuality' with sub-categories of autonomy, self-worth, private space, personal possessions, and finances, although nurses mentioned autonomy issues such as control over decisions more than residents did. The authors found that there were different emphases in residents' and nurses' responses. Residents mentioned specific physical functioning such as adequate eyesight and ability to walk as important to good quality of life, but implied that physical functioning alone was less important if they were philosophical or emotionally and spiritually content. The finding is consistent with other research which has shown that residents and nurses place different emphases on quality of life variables, prompting the fear that if residents and nurses' perceptions differ then resident needs may not be adequately met.

Residents' perceptions of quality of life were gathered by face-to-face interviews in 17 assisted-living facilities in the US (Ball et al., 2000). Fourteen significant domains of resident quality of life were identified by qualitative analysis of their responses. The five most significant domains were: psychological well-being, independence and autonomy; social relationships; meaningful activities; and care from the facility. Despite 94 per cent of sampled residents feeling very or somewhat satisfied with the care they received, feelings of depression and loneliness were expressed by more than half, and over one-third experienced anxiety and some boredom. Lack of independence, autonomy and choice were mentioned by the majority of sampled residents, and having something meaningful to do was an important part of residents' quality of life. The authors found that a key consideration in residents' quality of life was the 'goodness of fit' between the resident and the facility's social and physical environment. This increased when residents and their families had sufficient knowledge about what the facility offered in relation to residents' own needs, thus emphasising the necessity for prospective residents to plan ahead, and for facilities to provide clear information about their services, amenities and philosophy of care.

A similar study examining the quality of life of older people in assisted living facilities in the US found that a cohesive social environment, social participation and family involvement were associated with improved quality of life (Mitchell and Kemp, 2000). The study used measures of life satisfaction, social environment, depression and 'facility satisfaction' and also rated residents' levels of dependency, family contacts, social activities and opportunities for resident autonomy. They found that family contact and social activity participation were associated with higher life satisfaction. Overall, better quality of life was associated with a 'cohesive' environment (one in which staff or residents were more helpful and supportive of each other), participation in social activities and more contact with family. Indeed, participation in social activities was found to be predictive of better life satisfaction and low depression scores. They suggest that a living environment with less conflict, in addition to family and social involvement for residents are important for good quality of life in residential care.

Residents have also identified activities outside the home as important for good quality of life. A social services funded project, which had as one of its objectives to inform the contracting and purchasing process, was carried out to ascertain residents' views obtained from focus groups (Raynes, 1998). One feature of a good care home was identified as the opportunity for getting out of the home to go to a shop, a park, or to a class, for a walk, or to get a change of scene. A positive outcome of this project, following the distribution of the summary report to homes within the social services boundary, was the purchase of a minibus by one home to transport residents, and employment of 'leisure therapists' to promote resident activities. An important goal of this project was to involve and promote the views of the residents, thus making the services purchased on their behalf, related to their needs.

A comparative study (Shepherd et al., 1996) of community residential homes and long-stay hospital wards was carried out with a sample of adult psychiatric patients to measure quality of physical environment, management regimes, resident satisfaction and staff stress. Researchers assessed physical aspects of the homes and their 'general atmosphere' and used the Quality of Interaction Schedule (Dean et al., 1993), a non-participatory observation method recording and coding all interactions involving residents and staff. Resident satisfaction was assessed using the Lancashire Quality of Life Profile (LQOLP, Oliver et al., 1996). Hospital in-patients scored lower on measures of functional ability and were less likely to comply, while staff–resident interactions were less positive than in other settings. There were problems with missing data with the LQOLP, with just 22 per cent of the hospital sample completing the full interview, compared with 60 per cent in the residential homes, giving rise to concern that this could underestimate levels of dissatisfaction especially among hospital patients. Although the study was not carried out with older people, it is relevant since the authors concluded that use of conventional questionnaires or interviews may underestimate levels of dissatisfaction. They reported that judgements about life situations are made in subtle and complex ways and it may not be appropriate to use summary scores to report complex quality of life judgements, especially with the most disabled clients.

Observation studies in long-stay elder care settings have also been used, reportedly because of their unobtrusive nature (Clark and Bowling, 1990; Bowling and Formby, 1992). These studies looked at long-stay wards as an example of institutional life and also looked at activity in terms of disengagement theory. Patients were randomised to one of two nursing homes or to a geriatric ward. Assessments included measures of functional ability, mental orientation and confusion, life satisfaction and morale, and assessment of their quality of life in terms of their environment, meals, choice, privacy, relationships with others, and activities. The observation study was aimed at documenting activities and quality of everyday life in the three settings.

There were no differences found between the settings in terms of functional or mental ability, life satisfaction, or respondents' feelings about privacy. There was reluctance to express criticism, possibly due to low expectations or fear of repercussions. Nearly two-thirds of all respondents in each setting said they did nothing but 'just sit' morning and afternoon. There were fewer activities in the ward than in the homes, although many patients from the ward made up for lack of activity when they went to the patients' club. The observation study showed that the hospital patients' club was very popular among those who attended and was the most positive and stimulating of all the settings.

The authors concluded that respondents wanted to take part in various activities, and that occupational therapy was valuable to them. The observational study had been sensitive enough to discriminate between ward and homes, the more positive environment being the homes and the patients' club. Their findings supported the value of older people's engagement in everyday activities and interactions. The authors stressed the importance of using multiple methods in such environments, so as not to rely solely on interviews and assessments of mental and physical abilities, and consequently to take as broad a view as possible of quality of life.

'Dementia Care Mapping' (DCM) has been used to attempt to discover more about the quality of life of older people with dementia living in long-term care facilities. This method was originally developed by the Bradford Research Group (Kitwood and Bredin, 1994, 1997) to gain an understanding of care practice from the point of view and personal experience of the person with dementia. It uses an observational rating of activity type and a rating related to well-being and ill-being. A study was carried out among the residents of six care facilities, all of whom had been diagnosed with dementia using standardised psychiatric assessment (Ballard et al., 2001a). Dementia Care Mapping was undertaken with half the sample in each facility. It was found that more severe dependency and the use of psychotropic drugs were associated with significantly worse well-being, less time engaged in activities and significantly greater social withdrawal. Although none of the most dependent individuals had good or very good 'well-being' and reduced levels of functioning were not associated with 'ill-being', the authors stress the need to improve staff interaction with individuals who have greater levels of impairment. The use of psychotropic drugs was associated with reduced quality of life, which, the authors suggest, requires a more focused prescribing policy.

In summary, a good deal of research has been devoted to the definition and measurement of quality in long-stay care. This has ranged from broad and comprehensive measurement packages looking at the characteristics of care homes, to those concentrating on particular aspects of institutional life using face-to-face interview or observational methods. It is apparent that a substantial number of older people admitted to residential and nursing homes are affected by psychiatric disorders such as dementia and depression, many of them remaining undiagnosed or untreated. There are a number of messages emerging from the studies of quality of life discussed in this chapter. Although its definition remains imprecise, quality of life is essentially multi-dimensional. Research has focused on both objective and subjective components of quality of life, and health-related quality of life scales that measure functional ability are problematic in their application to older people. There is plenty of scope for further research into quality of later life, in particular with people residing in long-stay care homes and with significant cognitive impairment. Reflecting this, the study described in this book adopted a multi-dimensional approach to the measurement of quality of life of residents living in care environments.

3 The Study Design and its Methods

In this chapter the study design, research methods and research instruments and fieldwork procedures are explained, and data analysis procedures are discussed.

The design

The aim of this research — to relate differences in resident outcomes to characteristics of the care provided — could only be met by a longitudinal study design. The study was designed to measure improvement, maintenance or deterioration over time in a cohort of residents, in terms of physical and mental functioning and quality of life. The cohort members were to be located in a variety of care environments so that any outcome differences found could be related to variation in environmental characteristics. They were also to be newly admitted at the time of baseline assessment so that in comparing the progress of cohort members the study would be comparing people with similar amounts of exposure to the care environment.

It was not practicable to design the study in accordance with the theoretical ideal. First, the ideal would have been to establish baseline data on residents immediately prior to admission, so that change in the outcome measures over the study period could be related as closely as possible to the effects of institutionalisation, controlling for pre-admission condition. This was quite impracticable because it would have required screening of a large population of older people in the community in order to follow up a small number who in the event were admitted to residential or nursing care — and indeed admitted to a home which had agreed to participate in the study. The best practical approach to the study of new admissions was taken, with baseline assessments being carried out within two weeks of admission to one of the study homes.

Second, the ideal would have been to follow up the progress of cohort members at regular intervals until death or departure from the study home. Again a judgement had to be made for practical reasons because this would have required an open-ended research funding commitment. It was considered that the period of one year would be long enough to show measurable change in the outcome factors and the original study plan provided for final follow-up at 12 months with an interim assessment six months after admission. In the event, for reasons which will become clear, the final follow–up assessments were carried out nine months after admission.

Third, the ideal would have been to study a randomly selected group of homes — either by constructing a stratified and/or clustered sample or by following pre-selected cohort residents into whichever home they happened to be admitted. This was not possible for two reasons. In the first place it would have been unsatisfactory to have cohort members scattered in very small numbers across a large number of homes — to attempt to relate individual outcome to organisational characteristics with one studied resident in each of several hundred homes would have made no sense, practically or statistically. Secondly the research team had to be allowed access to homes in order to do the work at all.

Most research studies in organisations of any kind are based on convenience samples, the ideal of random sampling rarely being possible where the power to give or withhold access lies with owners or managers. Only two large-scale studies of randomly sampled institutions for older people have been carried out in the UK (Gurland et al., 1979; Godlove et al., 1980; Willcocks et al., 1987) since Townsend's work was done in the late 1950s (Townsend, 1962). Since the late 1970s changes in long-term care provision mean that the majority of homes are now privately owned. It has always been necessary to take some trouble in negotiating access to institutions but the experience of researchers is that these problems are greater in privately owned establishments. To have attempted to draw a random sample would have been fruitless because access refusals would immediately have rendered the sample unrepresentative. For these reasons the sample of homes was obtained by inviting all homes in the study areas with 25 or more beds to participate in the study, and then negotiating access with as many as possible. This exercise and its results are described more fully below.

Three geographical areas were chosen for conduct of the study in order to include a varied population in terms of occupation, social class, rural or urban environment. These were South Manchester, South/Mid Cheshire, and Blackpool, Wyre and Fylde. The first is an area of city and inner suburb. The second is a mixed area containing agricultural land, small market towns, some of considerable affluence, together with towns which were formerly major centres of railway work and salt mining. The third is one of the country's most popular seaside retirement areas, but also includes a fishing port and a rural hinterland.

Calculation of the desired sample size involved a number of uncertainties. Conventional comparative group power calculations were of no value. The primary objective of the study was not investigation by means of representative sampling of the prevalence of medical or other conditions in a larger population but evaluation of outcome in relation to specified environmental circumstances. Initially the sample size was calculated so as to ensure that the primary outcome measures — of depression, cognitive impairment and dependency — would be estimated to an acceptably high degree of precision (Snedecor and Cochran, 1980). For this purpose acceptable precision was defined as 95 per cent confidence intervals extending no further than 5 per cent either side of the parameter estimate.

The objective of attempting to relate resident outcome differences to variations in care environment characteristics gave rise to two additional considerations. First, it was clear that serious distortion would be produced if there were only one or two people in any individual home. It was difficult to establish a sound basis for calculating the number required in each home in advance of collecting any data about their individual characteristics. A somewhat arbitrary decision was taken, therefore, to aim for at least ten studied residents in each studied home. Second, although the sample of homes would not be statistically representative of all homes in England, or even of all homes in the north-west, it was desirable to use a sufficient number of homes to produce variation in the care environment measures and to ensure a reasonable degree of generalisability. These sampling requirements had to be met in the context of the realities of home admission rates and the expected length of survival following admission.

Based on the best information available when the study was planned (North West Elderly Care Project, 1994) several calculations were made:

- that to ensure the total sample size of 400 residents available to be followed up at the end of one year would require initial interviewing of 600 new admissions;
- that homes with fewer than 25 beds would be very unlikely to have ten or more new admissions within the proposed 12-month baseline period;
- that depending on bed numbers, and thus likely turnover rate, the study would have to include about 40 homes to achieve the desired resident sample. This was considered a sufficient number of homes for reasonable generalisability.

Thus the study set out to recruit approximately 40 homes, each with 25 beds or more. This last requirement precluded any generalisability to smaller homes which, it was considered, might have distinctive characteristics. Within these study homes it was planned to interview all residents admitted within a 12-month baseline period, to see them within 14 days of admission and to follow them up by repeat interviews six and 12 months later.

As the study progressed it became necessary to make amendments to the sample size and design. Although it proved possible to recruit only 35 homes, slightly fewer than the original target, this number was considered sufficient to meet the generalisability requirement. During the year prior to the start of fieldwork these homes had, between them, admitted a total of 632 new residents. This figure, given by home managers with the benefit of hindsight, was a true figure for long stay admissions, excluding all residents who left or died very quickly. If admissions had continued at that rate there would probably have been sufficient to meet the target of 600 allowing for refusals.

However new admission studies do not work with an existing population but rely on creation of the population as the work progresses. In this case it became apparent within the first three months of fieldwork that admissions were not taking place at the rate which had prevailed in the previous year. This was particularly so in Manchester where the start of fieldwork coincided with severe financial retrenchment on the part of the local authority and consequent reduction in publicly funded home placements. Because of policy changes beyond the control of the study it was clear that the baseline interview target would not be met within the time available.

In response to this an alternative strategy was employed, involving extension of the 12-month baseline to 15 months, with the follow-up interviews five and nine months after admission. With a 15-month baseline it was predicted that between 300 and 350 residents would be interviewed, still well short of the original goal of 600. Moreover, since there was considerable admission rate variation between homes it was likely that in a number of them there would be fewer than the target of ten residents to interview at the final follow up.

The statistical implications of this were considered. It was assumed, as for the original sample size calculations, that estimates were to be computed across all subjects, ignoring between-home differences. In reality it was known that this was not the case and that the statistical evaluation would have to take proper account of the stratified nature of the sample and estimate between-home and within-home variation. The effect of this necessary assumption would be to underestimate precision levels to some (at that stage unknown) degree.

If the original goal of interviewing 600 new admissions had been achieved, the 95 per cent confidence limits for the various key outcome measures considered would have been fractionally under 10 per cent of the inherent standard deviation; thus the original precision requirements for this study had been high. It was calculated that the newly projected resident recruitment, reduced by one-third attrition before final follow-up would be 13 per cent of the inherent standard deviation. The depression measure was the only principal outcome measure for which precision, rising to fractionally above five per cent of the sample mean, might be significantly adversely affected. For the other outcome measures the loss of precision would be small.

Since the minimum of ten residents per home had been set somewhat arbitrarily it was considered that slight reduction from this number in some homes would not involve an unacceptable loss of precision. More conventional power calculations were brought into play in considering the minimum number of homes which could be used in the analysis. A major part of the statistical evaluation would concentrate on evaluating changes over time. The number of individual residents available would be sufficient to detect as statistically significant very small changes in subject-specific measures. Detecting differences in home-specific measures would, however, be much more difficult. It was calculated that a total of 20–25 homes would be sufficient to detect changes in home-specific measures of around 70–75 per cent of the inherent between-homes standard deviation with 90 per cent power in the case of statistically normally distributed measures and with 80–85 per cent power if the data required nonparametric analysis.

Methods

Research instruments used to measure individual resident characteristics

The research instruments used in this study are shown in Box 3.1 and are described in full below.

Box 3.1
Resident assessment measures used in the study

- Mini-Mental State Examination (MMSE)
- Abbreviated Mental Test Score (AMTS)
- Geriatric Depression Scale (GDS)
- Barthel Activities of Daily Living Index (Barthel)
- (Modified) Crichton Royal Behaviour Rating Scale (Crichton Royal)
- Health of the Nation Outcome Scale 65+ (HONOS 65+)
- Lancashire Quality of Life Profile — Residential (LQOLP-R)
- Spitzer Uniscale
- Geriatric Mental State Schedule (GMSS)

Cognitive functioning Cognitive function was assessed using the Mini-Mental State Examination (MMSE) (Folstein et al., 1975) and the Abbreviated Mental Test Score (AMTS) (Hodkinson, 1972, 1973). The MMSE is a widely used screening instrument which can be administered in around ten minutes, its 20 items together producing a maximum score of 30. The test measures orientation to time, orientation to place, language, attention, visual construction, registration and recall, and sub-scores may be used to reflect these specific domains of cognitive ability. The cut-points commonly used to classify levels of cognitive impairment are: 24–30: no impairment; 18–23: mild impairment; and 0–17: severe impairment (Tombaugh and McIntyre, 1992). The version of the MMSE used in this study closely followed the original, with interviewees asked to spell 'world' backwards instead of doing the serial sevens test and in the recall task to recall the words 'apple, penny, table'.

The MMSE is a valid and reliable cognitive screening instrument which has been used in previous studies of nursing and residential home residents. Reported levels of short test-retest reliability have recorded reliability coefficients between 0.80 and 0.95 (Tombaugh and McIntyre, 1992). Braekhaus et al. (1992) reported good levels of validity on the total MMSE score (Pearson's r = 0.96). The majority of studies of dementia subjects have recorded sensitivity of the MMSE at around 87 per cent and positive predictive value of around 79 per cent, with greater sensitivity reported in studies including higher proportions of cognitively impaired subjects. Moderate to high levels of specificity have been recorded, although studies including psychiatric patients have reported lower levels (Tombaugh and McIntyre, 1992). MMSE performance has been found to be influenced by education and social class (O'Connor et al., 1989).

There is evidence that using more than one cognitive function test improves agreement with more lengthy diagnostic schedules and the MMSE–AMTS combination suggested by Hooijer et al. (1992 a, b) was employed in this study. The AMTS is a derivative of the Blessed Information, Memory and Concentration Test (Blessed et al., 1968), which has been validated against clinical and pathological diagnoses. It comprises ten items with a maximum score of 10 and a conventional cut-point for cognitive impairment of 7/8 (Hodkinson, 1972). Qureshi and Hodkinson (1974) reported acceptable levels of inter-rater reliability.

Depression The Geriatric Depression Scale (GDS) (Yesavage et al., 1983) was used as a screening instrument for depression. This extensively used instrument has the advantage of placing less emphasis than other rating scales on somatic symptoms, which are more likely in older people to be present for reasons other than depression. It is straightforward to administer, the questions requiring a simple yes/no response. The original GDS contained 30 items, but shortened versions have been produced (Yesavage, 1988) and the

15-item version was used in this study. This shortened version of the GDS has been found to correlate well with syndromal depression in a sample of older medical outpatients (Neal and Baldwin, 1994), with a score of over 5 on the GDS-15 being conventionally used to indicate depression 'caseness' (Yesavage, 1988). The individual GDS-15 items were found by D'Ath et al. (1994) to be associated significantly with total score and 'caseness'; indeed within the same study, 84 per cent of cases were identified by the single question, 'do you feel that your life is empty?'

There is some evidence that people who suffer from depression may perform badly on cognitive tests: 'As depression is known to be accompanied by intellectual disturbances in some cases, short dementia tests are known to risk false positive scores for dementia in cases of depression. The proper procedure would seem to be to use dementia and depression scales together' (McWilliam et al., 1988, as cited by Hooijer et al., 1992a). In spite of this, many studies have excluded subjects with low MMSE scores from assessment of depression (for example McCrea et al., 1994). In order to investigate the extent to which responses to depression questions could be obtained from cognitively impaired people the GDS-15 was administered in this study without any such prior selection.

In order to provide a check on the quality of the data produced by these short screening instruments, a sample of residents was interviewed within six weeks of admission using the Geriatric Mental State Schedule (GMSS) (Copeland et al., 1976). This standardised psychiatric interview has been used widely in studies of mental disorders in older people (for example Copeland et al., 1988). As well as its computerised diagnostic algorithm, AGECAT (Copeland et al., 1986) and History and Aetiology Schedule, it provides diagnoses according to DSMIIIR (the *Diagnostic and Statistical Manual*, third edition, revised) and ICD10.

Physical functioning To assess functional ability, behaviour and dependency, two measures were used — the Barthel Activities of Daily Living Index ('Barthel') (Mahoney and Barthel, 1965) and the Crichton Royal Behaviour Rating Scale — Modified Version ('Crichton Royal') (Wilkin and Thompson, 1989). Both were used in an informant interview with the key worker or other member of staff familiar with the resident. Assessments of functioning were based on what the resident actually did, rather than what the informant thought the resident capable of doing.

The ten scale items of the Barthel produce a maximum score of 20, with a lower score indicating greater dependency, and cover continence of bowels and bladder; personal grooming; toilet use; transferring; mobility; dressing; using stairs; and bathing. The best established and most commonly used dependency measure, the Barthel was described as 'the best buy amongst common ADL indices' by Collin et al. (1988). Novak et al. (1996) demonstrated that scores correlate well with the amount of time staff spend in providing care. Reliability (inter-rater and test-retest) has been tested in a range of settings using various methods of administration and found to be respectable (Wade and Collin, 1988). Some studies (for example Granger et al., 1979; Darton and Brown, 1997) have used three cut-points at 4/5, 8/9 and 12/13 to categorise levels of dependency. This method was used in this study, in addition to analysis based on the full score.

The Crichton Royal provides more specific assessment of dependency resulting from cognitive impairment. Originally designed for assessment of psychogeriatric patients, this scale has also been used in residential homes and hospital wards. Although it covers much of the same ground as the Barthel, the Crichton Royal adds items on orientation, communication, restlessness and memory and contains a Confusion Sub-scale which, with the cut-point of 4/5, has been shown by Vardon and Blessed (1986) to identify over 90 per cent of subjects with dementia. The complete scale's ten items give a maximum score of 38, with higher scores indicating greater dependency and/or more problematic behaviour. As with the Barthel, the scale has been found to correlate with the amount of staff time spent providing care (Evans et al., 1981). The cut-points of 1/2, 5/6, 10/11, 15/16 and 20/21 as used by Evans et al. (1981) were also used in this present study.

Quality of life Residents' quality of life was measured from several perspectives. The most important of these relied on the views of the residents themselves, obtained using an adapted version of the Lancashire Quality of Life Profile (LQOLP) (Oliver et al., 1996). Relatives' views on the quality of life of residents were sought using a postal questionnaire. The researchers' assessment was recorded using the Spitzer Uniscale (Spitzer et al., 1981).

The original LQOLP was developed for use with a younger population and had to be adapted for this study to improve relevance to elderly people in care homes. In the new version, the Lancashire Quality of Life Profile–Residential (LQOLP-R), questions relating to work, education and salary were omitted. Following pilot-testing some questions were re-worded and new questions were added concerning the home's food and occupational opportunities, based on the priorities of residential home residents expressed in Raynes' study (1995, 1996, 1998). The instrument contains some factual questions about marital status and family, hobbies and interests, but mainly consists of questions in the form 'How satisfied are you with [for example] the amount of privacy that you have here?' Single questions and sub-scales relate to particular life domains such as leisure, family relations, living situation and health and can be analysed separately as well as contributing to a global subjective well-being score. After pilot-testing, a 5-point 'Likert' scale was used for scoring levels of satisfaction or dissatisfaction rather than the 7-point scale used with younger respondents. The interview also contains the Bradburn

Affect Balance Scale (Bradburn, 1969) and the Rosenberg Self Esteem Scale (Rosenberg, 1965), in the version modified by Franklin et al. (1986). It concludes with a modified version of Cantril's ladder (Cantril, 1965), a global measure of life-satisfaction, in which respondents are required to rate their present lives by making a cross on a picture of a ladder. On the basis of pilot-testing experience with elderly home residents, the wording at the top and bottom of the ladder was modified to avoid the original's requirement to consider life in relation to the best or worst outcomes, which could have been expected at some unspecified period of life. In this study the ladder's extremes represented 'Life is as good as it could possibly be' / 'Life is as bad as it could possibly be'. Respondents were asked to mark a cross on the ladder to represent their current situation.

Because it was expected that a number of residents would be unable to understand the quality of life questions it was decided that the MMSE would be used to screen out those who were too cognitively impaired to do the LQOLP-R. It was originally anticipated that the LQOLP-R would be attempted only with residents who scored 16 or more on the MMSE but pilot-testing revealed that most residents who scored at least 10 were capable of understanding and answering at least some of the quality of life questions. In order to use this opportunity to test the MMSE as a screen for LQOLP-R 'interviewability' and to measure subjective quality of life for as many residents as possible, it was decided to reduce the threshold cut-point to 9/10.

The questionnaire for the relatives was designed for the study, and drew on various sources of which the main one was a study of quality measures in residential homes, carried out at the Institute of Psychiatry (Schneider et al., 1997a, b, c). The Raynes (1995) study identified other items which were included in the questionnaire. Relatives were asked, for example, whether they thought the resident had enough to do in the home, or enjoyable food. Relatives were asked to rate their overall satisfaction with the home and its services. They were also invited to record any comments they wished to make about the home, whether favourable or otherwise.

An interviewer-rated quality of life scale was included to record researchers' impressions of individual residents' quality of life, based on their knowledge following the direct and informant interviews. The Spitzer Uniscale (Spitzer et al., 1981) is a linear analogue scale which requires researchers to make a mark on a horizontal bar and is scored by measuring the distance of the mark from the end of the bar. This was used in work on the original LQOLP (Oliver et al., 1996), and shown to be significantly correlated with global well-being measures obtained from respondents.

A global outcome measure: the HONOS-65+ This instrument is based on the original HONOS, or Health of the Nation Outcome Scale, a mental health outcome scale developed by the Research Unit of the Royal College of

Psychiatrists (Curtis and Beevor, 1995; Wing et al., 1998) to measure a government defined target on mental health (Department of Health, 1992). The
HONOS has been shown to have good criterion validity and inter-rater reliability with a sample of older people with mental health problems (Shergill et
al., 1999). The large sample size of this study offered an opportunity to pilot
HONOS-65+ (Burns et al., 1999). The instrument was administered with the
Barthel and Crichton Royal as part of the informant interview. The interviewer's knowledge of the resident was used as well as that of the informant,
with the exception of the depression item where the informant's view was
recorded without interviewer input. The resident's mental or behavioural
problems over the preceding week were considered in each of 12 categories
and ratings were given on a scale from 0 (no problem), to 4 (severe problem).

Research instruments used to measure the characteristics of care

Physical environment Perhaps the most thorough and comprehensive attempt
to produce measurement instruments capable of collecting and evaluating
data across a wide range of institutions is the Multiphasic Environmental
Assessment Procedure (MEAP) developed over a number of years at Stanford
University's Center for Health Care Evaluation (Moos and Lemke, 1992). Two
instruments from this package were used in the study, one of them being the
Rating Scale which is designed for evaluation of residential institutions by
researchers, who rate what they see according to scoring guidelines given in
the instrument. It concentrates primarily (though not exclusively) on aspects of
the physical environment, including, for example, ratings of the neighbourhood, the grounds, attractiveness and cleanliness of the buildings, odour, condition of furnishings, the degree of variation or personalisation observed in
residents' rooms and so on. It is designed to be completed while making a tour
of the building but also requires the making of judgements about such matters
as staff availability to residents and organisation of the home. Since some of
these issues demand more than superficial acquaintance with a home, for this
study the Rating Scale was completed only after the researcher had visited the
home a number of times.

Social environment Both the instruments from the MEAP package were used to
assess characteristics of the social environment. The Sheltered Care Environment Scale (Moos and Lemke, 1984, 1992) is designed to measure various
attributes of the social environment by obtaining yes/no answers to 63 propo-
sitions. In this study it was given to staff as part of a questionnaire for anony-
mous self-completion. It contains seven sub-scales developed to measure
different dimensions of the social environment described by Moos and Lemke
as *Cohesion, Conflict, Independence, Self-disclosure, Organization, Resident influence*
and *Physical comfort.* In addition to the physical attributes mentioned above,

the Rating Scale allows researchers to rate the apparent level of activity in the home, physical and verbal interaction between staff and residents and the extent to which staff appear to be available to meet residents' needs. An additional global rating was added at the end of the Rating Scale, specifically for this study. Similar to an evaluation which relatives were asked to make of the homes when completing their questionnaires, it required allocation of the home to one of three categories, taking into account anything which seemed to the rater to be relevant:

A 'I would be happy to have a close relative living here and would feel reassured that the best possible care and quality of life was being provided.'
B 'I would have some reservations about having a close relative living here but think it would provide good enough care and quality of life to be acceptable if no better place was available.'
C 'I would not be at all happy about having a close relative living here.'

Public or private life Measurement of this aspect of life in the homes was inspired by the work of Willcocks et al. (1987). Homes appear to vary in the extent to which their residents lead what can be described as a predominantly 'public' life. In some homes residents appear to spend most of their time in their own rooms, emerging into communal areas only for meals; in others most residents appear to spend most of their time between meals sitting in communal lounges. Whether this apparent difference results from physical design or care practices such a difference in life style was considered to be of possible significance. A structured method of non-participant observation was devised, one purpose of which was to measure this dimension as one of the characteristics of care. Each home was toured eight times, starting on each hour between 10 a.m. and 5 p.m., with no more than four tours undertaken in any one home on the same day. Using a hand-held computer with a spreadsheet programme, for each resident observed in public space activity, location and verbal contact categories were coded. This enabled calculation of the proportion of the home's residents observed in public space. (For details of the observation method, see Appendix 1.)

Activity The other purpose of the observation study was to characterise the care environment in terms of the activity level of residents. As described above, the activities in which residents were engaged were recorded during the observation tours. This was used to produce a general activity breakdown and in particular to introduce to the analysis data on the proportion of resident observations classified as being without any apparent activity.

Home management and organisation Measurement of these characteristics was approached in various ways. Some basic information about the homes was obtained using a Home Preliminary Questionnaire distributed to all home managers prior to the start of fieldwork. This produced data on the home's size, sector and ownership, on staffing arrangements and on the charges made for care.

The nature of the home's management and the style of its leadership were investigated using interviews with the home owners or managers. These interviews were designed not only to collect information about the background, training and experience of those in positions of 'on site' leadership, but also to explore their ideas about the nature of leadership generally and the specific challenges of managing a care home for older people. In conjunction with these interviews a sample of staff were asked anonymously to complete versions of the Multifactor Leadership Questionnaire (Bass, 1985) to provide a 'follower's' view of the leadership they received.

The experience of being an employee in the home and the 'follower's' view of being led were also the subject of a number of scales in the Staff Questionnaire distributed to all staff working in the study homes. These were chosen from various sources and developed by workers at the University of Sheffield Institute of Work Psychology for a survey of mental health in the workforce of NHS Trusts (Borrill et al., 1996). These scales included eight measures of factors tested in the Sheffield study for their relationship to mental health. These were; *role ambiguity* (called *role clarity* in this study) (Rizzo et al., 1970), *role conflict* (Rizzo et al., 1970), *feedback* (Hackman and Oldham, 1975), *supervisory leadership* (Taylor and Bowers, 1972), *work demands* (Caplan, 1971), *social support at work* (West and Savage, 1988), *influence over decision making* (Borrill et al., 1996, from various sources) and *job autonomy and control* (Warr, 1990). High internal reliabilities and the psychometric adequacy of all these scales are reported by Borrill et al. (1996). In addition two organisational climate scales developed for the Sheffield study from the work of Lawthom, Patterson and West (1996) were included. Described as measures of *formalisation* and *autonomy* (called *initiative* in this study) they deal with the extent to which staff are controlled by rules and regulations or allowed to use their own initiative. To these was added a measure of *organisational commitment* (Cook and Wall, 1980).

Job satisfaction and staff mental health These were considered to be significant care characteristics in their own right, to be viewed separately from the management and leadership issues referred to above, as well as in conjunction with them. The Staff Questionnaire contained the 12-item version of the General Health Questionnaire (GHQ-12) (Goldberg and Williams, 1988) and a Job Satisfaction Scale (Warr et al., 1979). The former is a well established instrument widely used in screening for mental distress in normal populations, and for which its authors report six independently conducted validity studies which give median sensitivity and specificity for the measure of 86 per cent and 80 per cent respectively (Goldberg and Williams, 1988). The Job Satisfaction Scale is a 16-item scale covering a range of job issues including pay, hours, co-workers, superiors, job variety and responsibility, promotion opportunities and job security. Respondents are asked to rate their satisfaction with each of these aspects of working life on a 7-point 'Likert' scale.

Staff ratio As part of the Home Preliminary Questionnaire a complete list of staff names was obtained with job titles and normal weekly hours worked. Staff ratio calculations were done using this information. Details of staff sickness absence rates were also obtained. The *effective* staff ratio was difficult to calculate and interpret and was subject to distortion because of sickness and holidays, so an additional question was included. Managers were asked to give, in relation to the day on which they were completing the questionnaire, figures for the number of staff in various grades who were actually working at regular specified times throughout the day.

Staff qualifications, experience and in-service training In order to characterise care environments in terms of differences in staff expertise and skill–mix, the Staff Questionnaire asked staff to provide: information about the length of their experience in work similar to their present jobs; their qualifications; and any training they had received.

Casemix Although the study would collect very detailed information about the new admission cohort, the general level of dependency of the whole resident population in the homes was considered to be an important environmental variable which should be brought into the analysis in order to characterise the care environment. The final section of the Home Preliminary Questionnaire was designed to collect some very basic data of this kind. It was simplified as much as possible but did require the person completing the questionnaire to consider each resident in turn rather than to give answers in terms of the number of people with a particular dependency need — piloting suggested that this produced more accurate data and was easier for home staff to do than to make separate head counts for each disability category. (This questionnaire is reproduced as Appendix 2.)

Costs and charges for care Various methods were used to compile information about the costs of and charges made for care in the studied homes. The first task was to attempt an estimate of the overall cost of operating each of the homes and of the comparative opportunity cost of the investment in this particular use. As a starting point, copies of annual accounts were requested. These were readily available for the local authority and former local authority homes but a number of private sector homes refused to supply this information. The major contribution which staff costs make to any such operation could be calculated for each home using two sources of information. Details of staff numbers, grades and hours worked were obtained using the Home Preliminary Questionnaire; the Staff Questionnaire provided information about rates of pay and pension, holiday and sick leave entitlements for staff.

Both because it is of interest in its own right and because it offered an alternative approach in the event that private home costs proved to be impossible to calculate, all homes were asked for details of their charges. The basis on which these charges were made was investigated — for example whether different charges were made for people with different levels of care need, or for different standards of accommodation. Homes were also asked whether some specific services were included in the standard charge.

In order to arrive at a more individualised picture of the costs of, or charges for care, details of resident-related costs were obtained in relation to each resident included in the baseline assessment. This involved examination of the home's records after the earliest of three dates — the end of the nine–month follow-up period, the resident's death or departure from the home. By collecting information about services received during the relevant care period — visits from GPs, district nurses and other health professionals, out-patient care, special equipment provided — it was hoped that it would be possible to include in the costs assessment the significant factor of community health service provision.

Fieldwork

Any sizeable research project conducted outside a laboratory has to negotiate administrative hurdles and encounters various problems and challenges as the fieldwork progresses. Often these are not considered worth reporting but contain lessons that are useful, at least to others who are contemplating similar work.

The first task to be faced by this project's research team was the matter of obtaining local ethics committee approval. The study areas were chosen to represent a mixture of different types of population but the boundaries of the three chosen areas of South Manchester, South Cheshire, and Blackpool, Wyre and Fylde were drawn in terms of the geographical coverage of ethics committees. The project began before any arrangements were made for special ethics committee treatment of multi-centre studies and it was desirable to limit the number of separate applications for ethical approval to three. Nevertheless the process of obtaining approval of all three committees took several months. Their concerns differed in extent and subject matter, but in all cases it was necessary to establish acceptable protocols for obtaining participants' consent.

This is bound to be an issue in any research that involves a population including a significant proportion of cognitively impaired people, even where, as in this study, no treatment intervention is proposed. The consent protocol which was used by researchers for the study is reproduced as Appendix 3. The key principle was that no pressure or subterfuge should be used to persuade residents to participate and that interviews should be terminated if they changed their minds, or became too tired or distressed to continue.

The process of obtaining access to homes to do the research involved negotiation at more than one level. Lists of homes were obtained from local authorities and inspection teams and contact was made with local authority managers, the central managers of companies with several homes and with local organisations representing home operators. Letters of invitation were sent out to all (147) homes in the study areas with at least 25 beds, including residential and nursing homes in the private, voluntary and local authority sectors. Single page information sheets about the project and details of all personnel involved in it were sent with these letters, together with reply slips and prepaid envelopes. The approach of the letter was to invite those who might be interested to indicate that interest so that a visit could be made by appointment to discuss the matter personally with the manager. About half the homes approached in this way returned their reply slips with a 'yes' or 'no' response. Those who responded with a clear 'no' were not approached further. Homes which were equivocal or failed to respond at all were telephoned. These telephone discussions produced a number of opportunities to visit managers as well as some refusals. All the homes where managers were prepared to consider participation were visited so that the implications of the study could be discussed in detail and any questions answered. There were very few refusals at this stage. Some homes were unwilling to provide information about their costs and were included on that understanding.

Few research projects in care homes require the maintenance and nurturing of as many working relationships with staff as did this one. Unlike in cross-sectional studies, researchers did not arrive, spend time in the home interviewing people and then depart. Instead they were in and out of the homes on numerous occasions over a period of two years. During this time some staff left and new relationships had to be established. The team made a commitment to the homes to be as little trouble to them as possible — clearly it is not desirable for research workers to create disruption and extra work. However, a certain amount of imposition on the time and goodwill of staff was inevitable. In the vast majority of the homes working relationships were good throughout the project, indeed many staff were exceptionally welcoming and seemed to feel a sense of involvement with the research.

There was a very small number of homes in which it proved difficult or impossible to enlist the support and co-operation of staff for the project. Although on a day-to-day basis problems manifested themselves in the behaviour of more junior staff, this was invariably attributable to the manager's attitude to the research. In one home there appeared to be resentment by local management about central (i.e. off-site) management's agreement to participate in the study, which was conveyed through all levels of staff, leading to difficulties for quite some time.

During the six months prior to the start of the fieldwork programme the various instruments to be used were grouped into questionnaires and interview schedules which were printed on different coloured paper for ease of identification. The Screener, LQOLP-R and Informant Interviews were designed to be administered three times — within two weeks of admission, and on two follow-up visits. All residents were interviewed using the Screener, which contained the combined MMSE/AMTS and the GDS-15. On the back of this schedule was the Uniscale, to be completed by researchers at the end of the assessment, so that it would be based on maximum knowledge of the resident from direct interview and informant sources. The LQOLP-R was, as described above, administered only to those residents who scored 10 or more on the MMSE. The Informant Interview contained the Barthel, the Crichton Royal and the HONOS-65+. It also included a few general health questions that were symptom based rather than functional ratings and provision for listing details of diagnosed medical conditions and current medication.

The Home Preliminary Questionnaire, the Staff Questionnaire, the Rating Scale and two versions (initial and follow-up) of the Relatives' Questionnaire were also prepared and printed at this time. The Geriatric Mental State Schedule was used directly from a lap top computer. Standard documents and information sheets were prepared for the project: information for residents' general practitioners, to be sent with a standard letter, information for staff, and a larger print information sheet for residents and relatives. The consent form had project information printed on the reverse and a copy of this was left with residents at the time of first interview. Posters were produced for display in the homes, as were acetated copies of the project information and adhesive labels showing project contact details. Large numbers of Freepost envelopes were printed.

This project was sufficiently complex to require some care to be taken about its administrative procedures and the running of the office base. Several databases were set up, using Microsoft Access software. The most important of these was the resident database on which was recorded the resident's name, date of birth and admission (and death, when this occurred) as well as the name and address of the GP and nearest relative or friend. As the study progressed, the dates on which the various interviews were carried out were inserted and the progress of relatives' questionnaires and reminders was tracked. Systems were set up to notify researchers of follow-up interviews due, to prevent further approaches being made to residents who had declined further contact and to prevent questionnaires being sent to relatives when residents had died. This database, which was kept secure and confidential, provided the only link between residents' names and the numbers which were the only means of identification used on the interview schedules. To ensure that researchers would have available all the information they might require while out doing fieldwork, a Study Manual was prepared and supplied in loose-leaf binders so that updating could be carried out and additional sections inserted as required. It contained details of all project procedures — when and how contacts were to be made with homes or residents, how the study was to be explained, how consent was to be obtained and interviews carried out. It contained a flowchart of the interviewing process and a note on ethical guidelines and confidentiality. All the measurement instruments were described and detailed coding guidance was given, both to enable decisions to be made during interview and to standardise practice in areas where codes had to be allocated after the event. It also included a list of all contact names, addresses and telephone numbers of homes in the study as well as the home identification codes to be used.

During the preparatory phase, interview procedures were tested and the research team was trained, using the Study Manual, in the use of the research instruments by means of interviewing residents in a home used only for this purpose. In addition to classroom training sessions researchers carried out joint and co-rated interviews, the results of which were discussed and compared in order to achieve inter-rater reliability. The Study Manual provided a reference source throughout the project, helping to minimise researcher 'drift' and also constituted a permanent record of the study's procedures.

All the homes which had agreed to take part were visited about one month before new admission referrals were due to start being made to the study (1 September 1996). Managers were supplied with a folder containing materials which they would need — supplies of information sheets to be given to residents, relatives and staff; a supply of New Admission Forms for use when notifying the study team of a new arrival, by telephone or fax; posters about the study for display in the home; and adhesive labels with the study office address, telephone and fax number for attaching to telephones, admission books, computers, or wherever they would serve as a reminder. At the same time the manager was given a Home Preliminary Questionnaire with a Freepost envelope for its return.

Homes were asked to telephone or fax the project office with details as soon as a resident was admitted, or indeed a few days beforehand if the admission had definitely been arranged. This was sometimes forgotten and some new admissions were notified too late to be included in the study. To ensure that this happened as little as possible, homes were telephoned every one to two weeks throughout the 15-month baseline period. When referrals were taken, home staff were reminded to tell residents and/or relatives that the home was taking part in the study and to give them copies of the project information for residents and relatives. This was given only to relatives in cases where the resident had severe memory loss or was thought to be so anxious that advance notice of the arrival of a strange researcher would exacerbate anxiety.

On receipt of referral details a letter was sent to the resident's GP, enclosing information about the study and asking the GP to telephone the project office in the event of there being medical reasons indicating that the resident should not be interviewed. This resulted in a very small number of enquiries but only one objection to inclusion of a patient. After the time period for GP objections had elapsed a researcher made arrangements to visit the resident in the home. In a small number of cases the home manager or a relative felt strongly that the resident should not be approached, usually because of serious or terminal physical illness. With those exceptions a researcher saw all referred residents. Even in cases where home staff said 'you won't get anything sensible out of him ...' it was the policy of the research team to make a direct approach to the resident. Thus wherever possible refusals were received directly and researchers did not rely on the views of intermediaries.

The study was designed to investigate the outcome of long-term care but the distinction between long and short-term is often difficult to define in practice. During the first few weeks of fieldwork it became apparent that this was causing a problem. The staff of the study homes had been asked to refer all new admissions intended to be for long-term care, and also any which were nominally short-term but where all concerned expected a long-term arrangement to ensue. In order to have a workable operational definition it was stated that the study would include all admissions made without a definite discharge date specified on admission. This quickly proved to be unworkable because in some of the homes almost all admissions were defined as short-term, with pre-arranged discharge dates, and then converted into long-term. This may have been due to a desire to give formal status to a trial period of residence; it may also have been related to the higher weekly rate of payment received from the local authority for care defined as short-term. Whatever the reason, this resulted in several new admissions being missed in the very early weeks of fieldwork. This was rectified by a procedural change so that all admissions were notified which were either:

- explicitly long-term;
- short-term with the resident also on a waiting list for long-term care; or
- short-term but resident considered by manager to be 'almost certain' to stay for long-term care.

This changed definition worked reasonably well but was not perfect and it is possible that the admission period is so full of uncertainty that no such definition will fit all circumstances. A resident admitted with the express intention of having two weeks' post-operative convalescence can deteriorate and decide that long-term care is necessary. A resident admitted for respite while caring relatives take a holiday may find that the relatives use the holiday to review the nature of their caring commitment.

The study's consent procedures worked reasonably well although there were borderline situations which were difficult to decide how to handle. Many residents were quite able to understand what was involved and to give their own consent. This included many of those who were cognitively impaired. A degree of disorientation (particularly perhaps in newly admitted people) or of memory loss is not incompatible with being able to make a decision about answering research questions. It was not unusual for residents to say things like 'I've got a terrible memory — I don't know whether I'll remember what you've said two minutes after you've said it but I'm quite willing to have a go'. Staff were asked to witness consents in cases where researchers were unsure about whether or not the explanation had been understood, and asked to consent by proxy where there was even less confidence in their understanding but the resident gave no sign of objecting to the interview.

The last situation is of course problematic but to have no such procedure would have meant automatic exclusion of everyone with severe dementia. Since no study of long-term care outcome could proceed sensibly while ignoring people with that disability it was considered justifiable to thus extend the consent arrangements. It was relevant to this that the study did not involve any treatment or drug administration, nor was the interviewee's place of residence or the care received affected in any way by it. Some interviews were terminated after a few questions when the resident appeared to become anxious or distressed and some residents asked to stop half way because they felt too tired to continue. On other occasions the researcher decided to stop because the resident appeared so ambivalent about participation that refusal had to be assumed.

It is unlikely that any consent protocol would fit all cases and avoid all dilemmas. Ultimately any procedure has to be interpreted and applied and the spirit of the interpretation is of major importance. The overriding concern in this project was that residents should not be induced to participate by pressure of any kind or by subterfuge, including allowing any misunderstandings to persist that interviewers were providers of care or treatment or would help them in some way. These principles guided researchers in their interpretation of the rules and the fact that a significant number of people did refuse is seen as evidence that this approach was effective.

Some care was taken to achieve conditions which would be conducive to a successful interview. It was treated as an absolute rule that interviews could not take place with anyone else in the room. Usually residents were happy to be interviewed in their own rooms; in other cases small lounges and corners of unused dining rooms were used. Doors were closed, with the explanation given to residents that it was necessary to speak privately and not within the hearing of others. This was used to reinforce the assurance of confidentiality which formed part of introducing the study. Residents were always addressed using their surnames and care was taken to maintain the respectful demeanour appropriate to the circumstances.

On occasion it was not possible to speak to residents alone because they refused to be separated from the company of others. A few married couples who had been admitted to care together were excluded from the study for this reason. If relatives or other visitors were present researchers would wait or return another day; this was also done with residents who were reluctant to move from the lounge to a private room but would be interviewed before leaving their rooms in the morning. Residents with hearing impairment were interviewed with the aid of a *Sarabec* communicator which occasionally resulted in dramatically improved quality of communication. A number of such residents had no hearing aids — for one man it was clear that this equipment enabled him to hear a human voice for the first time in many years — or refused to use them because of background noise. For an interview where 'one to one' communication is desired, to the exclusion of other sounds, this equipment seems to give superior results.

The actual interviewing procedure was similar on all three visits to the resident. The Screener interview was done first and if the resident scored 10 or over on the MMSE this was followed by the LQOLP-R. These interviews took, on average, 19 minutes and 28 minutes respectively but this varied enormously. Interviews were sometimes very long because it was difficult to keep the interviewee 'on task'. Some interviewees simply wanted to talk and expanded on every aspect of the interview. After such interviews it was often the case that the researcher would be thanked — 'it's been so nice to have someone to talk to like this' — but on one memorable occasion the interviewer emerged after a marathon session dominated by the resident's verbosity only to overhear as she left, 'That woman's kept me talking for ages; she kept asking me all these questions'.

The Informant Interviews were usually done after the resident interview or after all residents for interview in the home on that day had been seen. Occasionally it was necessary to return at a less busy time. The informant would be the key worker or other member of staff who knew and cared for the resident.

GMSS interviews were carried out once only with a sub-sample of residents. Alternate residents who were screened within 14 days of admission were approached for this purpose within one month of the Screener interview. Unlike the other interviews for which paper schedules were used, they were done using a lap top computer into which data was entered directly as the interview progressed. To avoid contamination they were undertaken by an interviewer who was blind to the previously completed resident and informant interviews, instructions being prepared by the project secretary using forms which provided essential contact information only. Questionnaires for relatives were prepared in two versions; the one used for the two follow-up distributions omitted questions about the admission process and personal data about the responding relative. Although called the 'Relatives' Questionnaire' this was designed not for the formal next of kin but for regular visitors who in some cases were friends rather than relatives. The name and address of the most involved relative or friend at the time of admission was obtained and the questionnaires were sent out three times, shortly after each of the three visits to residents. Freepost envelopes were supplied for their return and reminder postcards went out a month after the original questionnaire if it had not been returned by then.

The postal questionnaire given to all staff was administered once, during the first six months of the fieldwork period accompanied by a programme of presentations given at staff meetings to encourage participation. Subsequently, a prize draw was carried out to reward participants. Freepost envelopes were supplied for return of the questionnaires and, as with the relatives' questionnaire, reminder postcards were despatched after one month.

Researchers completed the Rating Scale for each home once during the fieldwork period, the only requirement for the timing of this being that they had visited the home on a sufficient number of occasions to feel familiar with it. The individual costs data were collected toward the end of the fieldwork period so that this could be done in relation to the full nine months for all residents followed up for that period. The observation study data collection was conducted over a period of approximately eight months in the middle of the two-year fieldwork period. It was arranged so that observation sessions could be done on days when researchers were visiting homes in order to do interviews.

Analysis

The main purpose of this study was to investigate relationships between change in residents' well-being over time and variables representing aspects of the 'care environment', and this was the focus of the main, longitudinal analysis. However, aspects of the data were subjected to separate, additional analyses. The data collected about the homes and about the residents within two weeks of admission were analysed as a cross-sectional survey to give a description of this large cohort of new admissions and the care being provided for them. Data from the staff questionnaire were analysed independently as a major survey of care home staff, their pay, conditions of service and work circumstances. Data from the measures used to assess cognitive impairment, depression and quality of life were also used for specific work aimed at contributing to methodological development.

A wide range of statistical methods was, therefore, used to examine the data in different ways. Parametric and non-parametric techniques such as chi-square, t-tests and Mann-Whitney statistics were calculated in order to consider differences between two groups (such as nursing compared with residential homes, survivors compared with those who died) and analysis of variance for comparisons between groups of three or more. Parametric (Pearson's r) and non-parametric (Spearman's rho) correlation coefficients were used to consider the linear relationships between continuous variables. In each case parametric tests were used when the data allowed. Otherwise non-parametric equivalent tests were used. Principal Components Factor Analysis and Cluster analysis (K-means clustering with classification and iteration) were used to analyse the data from the staff-completed Sheltered Care Environment Scale.

As part of the main longitudinal analysis, Cox regression analyses were run on the survival data to identify variables that contributed to the likelihood of survival. Survival analysis concerns the time until a specified event occurs, in this case death. Cox's proportional hazards regression model allows the investigation of the effect of a number of variables on survival (Cox and Oaks, 1984). For this study, survival time was calculated as the length of time (in days) from admission until the calculation point 290 days after data collection began, or death, which ever was the sooner. The censoring variable was death. Some residents left the homes or refused further contact during the period of the study. Data pertaining to this small group were included by calculating their survival time until the period when contact ceased. One of the strengths of this type of analysis is that such cases are included in the analysis. Data augmented by additional follow-up data, collected about one year after the end of the study period were also used to identify factors that contributed to the likelihood of survival.

Multiple Linear Regression and Logistic Regression were used to analyse the impact of features of the care environment on the various outcomes for residents. Multiple Linear Regression estimates the coefficients of the linear equation (involving one or more independent variables) that best predict the value of the continuous dependent variable. Logistic regression is a similar technique where the dependent variable is dichotomous rather than continuous.

In summary

- The study was conducted in 35 residential and nursing homes, each with 25 beds or more, located in three geographical areas of north west England.

- Newly admitted residents were interviewed within 14 days, using measures of cognitive functioning and a depression scale. Measures of resident's physical functioning, behaviour and dependency were completed by a staff member. Follow-up interviews were carried out at five and nine months following admission.
- A number of sampled residents were interviewed about their satisfaction with aspects of the home using an adapted version of the Lancashire Quality of Life Profile (the Lancashire Quality of Life Profile — Residential). Relatives were also sent questionnaires to gain their views of the home.
- Basic information about each home was obtained and in-depth interviews were conducted with home owners or managers to gain information about resident-mix, management and leadership style. The characteristics of the care environment were rated by researchers.
- Questionnaires were distributed to each home for completion by all members of staff. The staff questionnaire contained a number of well-validated scales and was designed to gather a range of views on the care environment and on the experience of being an employee in the home.
- A Study Manual was developed to provide details of administrative, consent and interview procedures. This provided a source of reference throughout the project and a permanent record of study procedures.
- A range of statistical methods was employed to examine the data including parametric and non-parametric tests. Survival data were analysed using Cox regression and Cox's proportional hazards regression. Features of the care environment and resident outcome were analysed using multiple linear and logistic regression.

4 The Homes, the Residents and their Daily Lives

This chapter examines the characteristics of the homes in the study, their staffing, resident mix and attributes of quality. It then considers the individual residents included in the study, and provides more detailed information about their lives within the homes.

The homes

Some of the homes which agreed to take part did not, in the event, have enough new admissions during the 15-month baseline period to be included in the study. This was largely due to changes in local authority admission policies which occurred just as fieldwork began. Between the 12-month period prior to the start of the study and the first 12 months of fieldwork (i.e. between 1995/6 and 1996/7) the number of admissions to the original group of Cheshire study homes fell by 13 per cent, to Blackpool homes by 42 per cent and to Manchester homes by 58 per cent. This resulted in some homes contributing only one newly admitted resident to the study. Five homes were excluded because they contained very few study residents, leaving the final sample of 30 homes.

In Table 4.1 the 30 homes are compared with the 35 original participating homes and with all homes in the sampling frame (homes with at least 25 beds in the three study areas). Comparing the final sample to all homes in the sampling frame, private homes are under-represented to a statistically significant degree (χ^2 (2) = 12.08, p = 0.002). However 40 per cent of the homes were privately owned and the study probably included a greater number of such establishments than has ever been included in a UK study involving intensive interviewing. It included local authority homes, former local authority homes

49

Table 4.1
Size, ownership sector and type of care

	The 35 original homes	The 30 homes in the final sample	All homes in the three areas with at least 25 beds
Size (bed numbers)			
Min.	25	27	25
Max.	125	125	150
Median	35	39	35
Sector (number of homes)			
Private	17 (48.6%)	12 (40%)	106 (72.1%)
Voluntary/former local authority	12 (34.3%)	12 (40%)	24 (16.3%)
Local authority	6 (17.1%)	6 (20%)	17 (11.6%)
Type of care (number of homes)			
Nursing beds only	15 (42.8%)	11 (36.7%)	73 (49.7%)
Residential beds only	18 (51.4%)	18 (60%)	66 (44.9%)
Joint registered homes	2 (5.7%)	1 (3.3%)	8 (5.4%)

devolved to voluntary sector ownership, independent non-profit homes, private homes managed by their proprietors and homes which were part of large companies operating many homes throughout the country.

The reduction in admissions had considerable implications for the homes themselves, as well as for this research project. Some of the homes included in the sample had low occupancy rates. Overall the median occupancy rate in July 1997 was 92 per cent in the Manchester homes, 89 per cent in the Cheshire homes and 77 per cent in the Blackpool area homes, but this conceals some very low individual figures — one home with 38 per cent of its beds occupied was probably operating at the very limit of financial viability.

Among the study homes a wide range of buildings and physical environments was represented. All the local authority and former local authority (now voluntary) homes were in buildings constructed within the last 40 years, were purpose built and either single or two storey. As buildings they were similar to thousands of other homes throughout the country, often built in a square or rectangular formation, with long corridors. The homes which were still in direct local authority ownership showed fewer signs of expenditure on modernisation or refurbishment than those transferred to the voluntary sector. The latter were, during the study, undergoing a major programme of refurbishment, from which they emerged, one by one, with new carpets, wallpaper, improved garden and courtyard areas and better office and reception facilities.

Single rooms for residents were the norm in these purpose built homes, with limited provision of double accommodation available for couples.

Although often quite pleasant and attractively decorated, these rooms were small and suitable for use as bedrooms rather than as bed-sitters. En suite toilet facilities were not available.

By contrast, all but three of the private homes and one of the 'non-group' voluntary homes were in buildings adapted from other uses. Usually they had been large private houses; most were built in the nineteenth century; one had been extensively adapted from a very old semi-industrial building. There was variation in the degree to which these buildings appeared suitable for their present purpose and in the quality of the adaptation. Some of these homes appeared to work well for residents and, having been equipped with lifts, ramps and mobility aids, offered a pleasant and usable environment with the benefits of somewhat larger rooms and attractive architectural features. However, double rooms were more common than in purpose built homes and there was some sharing between residents who met for the first time when asked to share a bedroom. In one home some residents had small and rather oppressive rooms in what had once been servants' quarters at the top of the building, with small windows which provided limited light or external view. Several of the adapted buildings also provided a tiring work environment for staff, particularly where nursing care was being provided. In some cases lifts were few, slow and tiny so that staff spent a good part of the day running up and down long flights of stairs. In others it was difficult to manoeuvre wheelchairs in narrow corridors.

The homes also varied in the extent to which residents, particularly those suffering from dementia, appeared to be able to find their way around. The purpose built homes were simpler in design and a number had the advantage that someone wandering along the corridor would, sooner or later, arrive back at the same place. However, rooms and doors in such buildings often appear very similar and signposting or room naming was not universally used. In some of the adapted buildings the rooms were more distinctive and signs were used; others seemed like mazes, even to researchers much younger than their residents and after repeated visits over a period of two years.

The study homes included examples of a variety of organisational structures. The local authority and former local authority homes were, of course, run as part of larger organisations, with, in both cases, on-site managers accountable to head office superiors. A similar managerial pattern prevailed in a number of the private homes, some of which were part of organisations operating a number of establishments throughout the country. On-site managers working within these structures had access to, or were required to use, head office services for such functions as accounting, purchasing and personnel management. As is invariably the case in large organisations the connection between on-site manager and head office function could be, depending on a number of organisational and personal factors, a benefit or a burden. Either way, it placed limits on the freedom of action, or 'position power' of the on-site manager.

By contrast, several study homes in the private sector were small independent businesses, owned and directly managed by single proprietors or partnerships, often by married couples or run as family businesses involving more than one generation. In these homes, the on-site manager, though subject to the usual external constraints affecting any business and to the requirements of inspection authorities, was entirely autonomous. As with the situation facing managers within larger organisations, this could be a blessing or a curse, depending on many circumstances. It was clear that these manager/proprietors valued their freedom of decision making, the ability to change in response to market demands or residents' wishes and the fact that they could hire and fire staff constrained only by law and their own morality rather than by personnel management procedures. When difficulties arose, however, they were on their own, without easy recourse to professional supervision and guidance, or to help in dealing with the exigencies of market forces.

Table 4.2 displays staff ratio calculations for different groups of staff, and enables comparison to be made between the nursing and residential homes. All the figures in this table refer to staff hours per occupied bed per day. No allowance is made for holidays or sick leave so that the time available is a somewhat generous estimate. Staff are grouped in various ways. 'Senior staff' is a grouping which includes all staff with supervisory or autonomous professional responsibility for resident care — managers, deputy managers, care supervisors and team leaders, qualified nurses and sisters. 'Care assistants' are all care or nursing assistants or nursing auxiliaries. The 'all carer' category is probably the best one for comparison between nursing and residential homes in that it includes all staff with direct caring responsibilities and contact with residents — nurses and sisters, care supervisors, care and nursing assistants.

Table 4.2
Hours of staff time available per occupied bed per day

	Mean	Std dev.	Min.	Max.
Nursing homes (12 homes)				
Senior staff (managers/nurses/supervisors)	1.29	0.40	0.74	1.83
Care/nursing assistants	2.50	0.52	1.69	3.47
All carers (nurses and assistants)	3.44	0.67	2.33	4.99
Domestic and catering	1.11	0.30	0.76	1.67
Residential homes (18 homes)				
Senior staff (managers/nurses/supervisors)	0.71	0.22	0.36	1.26
Care/nursing assistants	1.77	0.53	0.56	2.71
All carers (nurses and assistants)	2.07	0.57	0.56	2.96
Domestic and catering	0.80	0.25	0.40	1.27

As might be expected the staff ratio figures are higher in nursing than in residential homes, where a mean of just over two hours of 'all carer' time per occupied bed per day was available. The nursing home equivalent was 3.4 hours. There was, however, considerable variation within the nursing home and residential home groups. As the minimum and maximum figures show, in residential homes care assistant time per occupied bed per day ranged from just over half an hour, to nearly two and three quarter hours. In nursing homes 'all carer' time per occupied bed ranged from just under two and a half hours to under just five hours per day. Across both types of home the range for domestic and catering staff was from about 25 minutes to one hour 40 minutes per occupied bed per day.

By way of comparison, it is useful to note that Willcocks et al. (1987) reported staff hours available per resident day in the residential homes they studied as 0.44 hours for senior staff, 1.3 hours for care staff and 0.5 hours for domestic staff.

The figures in Table 4.3 represent the ratio of residents to all care staff at specific times during one particular day and provide further illustration of this variation between homes. To take some examples, at 5 p.m. on this one day, in the best staffed nursing home there were four residents to each member of the nursing or care staff compared with eight residents in the worst staffed nursing home. In the residential sector there were between five and 28 residents to each member of the care staff at 5 p.m.

Certain categories of staff were in short supply everywhere, but better represented in some homes than others. There were no designated activity

Table 4.3
Ratio of residents to all care staff at various times on one day

	Mean	Std dev.	Min.	Max.
Nursing homes (12 homes)				
Residents to all care staff 8 a.m.	4.44	1.01	2.16	5.88
Residents to all care staff 11 a.m.	4.54	0.71	3.6	5.88
Residents to all care staff 2 p.m.	4.73	1.46	2.08	6.67
Residents to all care staff 5 p.m.	6.03	1.06	4.2	8
Residents to all care staff 9 p.m.	8.39	1.42	6.67	10.5
Residents to all care staff 2 a.m.	10.33	3.69	6.75	21
Residential homes (18 homes)				
Residents to all care staff 8 a.m.	7.94	1.94	5.25	12.5
Residents to all care staff 11 a.m.	8.63	5.26	3.5	28
Residents to all care staff 2 p.m.	9.39	4.84	3.5	25
Residents to all care staff 5 p.m.	10.47	5.25	5.25	28
Residents to all care staff 9 p.m.	11.26	5.27	5.25	28
Residents to all care staff 2 a.m.	14.18	3.94	5.25	19.5

staff in 14 of the homes and only three homes had more than 25 hours per week of activity staff time. Eighty per cent of the homes provided less than six minutes of activity staff time per occupied bed per day. Administrative and secretarial staff were completely absent from 15 homes.

All but one of the 30 homes provided details of their weekly charges and of their public and private charging structure. These structures were very variable. For publicly funded residents dependency banding scales were applied in some homes but not others, depending on local authority practice. In a number of homes charges varied according to the quality of accommodation purchased — with or without en suite toilet facilities or full bathrooms, with or without balconies or terraces, according to the size of the room. Occasionally charitable funds were applied to support the care of voluntary home residents. In some cases charges to self-funding residents were, it appears, made on an ad hoc basis, according to a judgement of how much the market would bear. In 15 of the 29 homes for which charging information was obtained the minimum private charge was higher than the minimum publicly funded charge, by an average of £33 per week (range £10–£71 per week). Thus, in one home, a similar service to two residents in adjoining rooms with similar dependency needs would cost £71 a week more to a private paying resident than the local authority would pay for the other.

The impact of fixed prices by local authority purchasers was such that the weekly price variables are by no means normally distributed. In Table 4.4, in order to produce comparative data on minimum and maximum charges the dependency banding structure used by some homes was applied, as far as possible, to the others. Thus the local authority homes which provided residential care at one price regardless of dependency are treated as if they 'banded' residents — the three prices at which they would care for three differently disabled residents are identical. Taking charges to publicly and

Table 4.4
The homes' charges (£ per week, 1997 prices)

	Min.	Max.
Publicly funded residential care, low dependency	203	262
Publicly funded residential care medium dependency	211	262
Publicly funded residential care high dependency	228	287
Homes' lowest charges for private residential care	223	271
Homes' highest charges for private residential care	228	312
Publicly funded nursing care, low (nursing) dependency	304	330
Publicly funded nursing care, medium (nursing) dependency	307	330
Publicly funded nursing care, high (nursing) dependency	307	330
Homes' lowest charges for private nursing care	304	375
Homes' highest charges for private nursing care	304	500

privately funded residents into account, weekly charges for residential care ranged from £203 to £312 and for nursing care from £304 to £500.

Homes were asked about services charged as extras or which residents were expected to purchase directly from outside suppliers. Chiropody was an included service in 15 of the 30 homes (about equal proportions in the nursing and residential sectors). Physiotherapy was included by all but two nursing but by only four of the residential homes. All the nursing homes and most of the residential homes provided incontinence supplies without extra charge. Of the four residential homes where this did not happen, in three homes residents had to pay for their own supplies and in one these were provided free by the NHS. These variations were due, at least in part, to different arrangements made by the local authorities and NHS providers. Clearly these differentially influenced the costs to different local authorities and individual residents.

Using questionnaires in the form reproduced as Appendix 2, homes supplied information about all their residents — not just the cohort of new admissions included in the study. The questions covered a number of disability and dependency criteria and make it possible to see different 'casemix' patterns in the homes which are likely to have contributed to differences in the overall care environment. Homes provided information about all residents in occupation at the time of completing the questionnaire. This resulted in collection of data on a total of 1057 residents, of whom 507 were in nursing homes (including the one home with joint registration) and 550 in residential homes.

Table 4.5 illustrates the range of reported dependency. In relation to each of the specific dependency areas it shows minimum, median and maximum percentages for the two separate groups of residential and nursing homes. For example, among the group of residential homes the one with the lowest proportion of its population needing help with walking had 3 per cent of

Table 4.5
Percentage of each home's residents with specific dependencies

	Min. % res. home	Median % res. home	Max. % res. home	Min. % nursing home	Median % nursing home	Max. % nursing home
Unable to walk unaided	3.1	23.3	48.0	47.9	68.5	82.1
Unable to use wc unaided	0	21.3	37.5	19.4	57.2	92.6
Unable to feed unaided	0	6.5	17.6	4.9	16.5	33.3
Unable to wash unaided	0	24.8	60.0	24.3	53.9	89.6
Incontinent	6.1	27.2	46.7	21.1	42.6	78.9
Disoriented	16.7	39.7	63.6	31.6	49.4	94.4
Memory problems	14.3	46.7	75.0	31.6	58.3	94.4
Behaviour problems	2.8	13.8	78.9	4.9	25.1	58.3

residents dependent in this way; at the other extreme 48 per cent of another residential home's population were unable to walk unaided. For all the dependency criteria median percentages are higher in the nursing than in the residential homes but the differences appear to be somewhat less for those which are specifically concerned with mental incapacity. Median percentages in residential homes of 39.7 per cent for persistent disorientation and 46.7 per cent for persistent short-term memory problems were higher than in some of the nursing homes. Apart from the problem behaviour category, the homes with the maximum percentages of all these dependency needs among their residents are nursing homes.

Problem behaviour did in fact seem to be rather differently distributed. Of the four homes which reported that over 50 per cent of their residents had persistent behaviour problems, three were residential. The apparent lack of relationship between reported problem behaviour and disorientation or memory problems was also surprising. In one nursing home, for example, with 94.4 per cent of its residents described as disoriented and with memory problems it was reported that only 5.6 per cent manifested problem behaviours.

Rating the homes' environmental quality: the Multiphasic Environmental Assessment Procedure Rating Scale

The Rating Scale is one component of the MEAP used by Moos and Lemke (1992) to organise and record a researcher's rating of the quality of a care home environment, both physical and social. Completed by researchers after at least three visits to the home, it was scored and analysed using the instructions provided by its authors. It contains 24 items organised in four sub-scales measuring the physical attractiveness of the overall site and internal home environment; the extent to which the environment is diverse and stimulating; staff functioning; and resident functioning. Its authors report, on the basis of testing in 93 Californian facilities, high internal consistency (Cronbach's α = 0.82, 0.73, 0.82 and 0.67 for these four sub-scales respectively). Scoring is done so as to represent the percentage of total possible points awarded by the rater. For example, the Physical Attractiveness sub-scale comprises nine items, each carrying three points for a possible maximum score of 27. A home awarded 'full marks' for Physical Attractiveness (27 points) would be given a Rating Scale score of 100.

- *physical attractiveness of the overall site — neighbourhood, grounds and buildings assessed for maintenance, quality and general attractiveness*

None of the homes was considered to be in an unpleasant or unattractive neighbourhood and nine were given the highest neighbourhood rating of 'very pleasant'. Similarly most of the homes had attractive and reasonably or well maintained grounds or buildings, with only seven homes rated as 'unattractive' or 'ordinary'.

- *physical attractiveness of the four major living areas (lounges, dining rooms, hallways, bedrooms) assessed for noise, odours, quality of illumination, cleanliness, and condition of the interior and furnishings*

Predictably, public areas were noisier than private ones, lounges in 17 homes being rated as 'somewhat noisy' — which could have applied to a lively sound of conversation. None were 'very noisy'. In all but four homes the bedrooms were quiet. Most of the homes were free of objectionable odours; where these were noted, they were most often present in hallways (seven homes). While the majority of lounges and dining areas were considered to have good or adequate lighting, the hallways and bedrooms were relatively poorly illuminated — the hallways of ten and the bedrooms of more than half the homes had 'inadequate' or 'barely adequate' lighting. With only one exception the homes were reasonably clean, particularly in the public living areas. Bedrooms and hallways tended to be dirtier, with bedrooms in seven homes and hallways in six considered to be dirty.

In all areas except hallways the condition of walls and floors was reasonably good, in terms of holes in carpets, chips out of the walls and so forth. Over three-quarters of the lounges, dining areas and bedrooms had walls and floors of a good standard. Except in the bedrooms the standard of furniture was good, bedroom furniture being poor in one home and only fair in another ten.

- *diversity and stimulation — windows (adequacy of provision and view), variation and personalisation of residents' rooms, distinctiveness of living spaces*

Windows in most public areas were considered at least to be adequate, but there were 11 homes in which bedrooms were rated as having windows too few in number or too small. In many homes, views from the windows were dull or lacking in interest (lounges in 18 homes, hallways in 21).

In most homes residents' rooms showed some evidence of attempts to provide variation and personalisation. In public living spaces only one home was rated as 'institutional' in style and decor; in 12 homes a concerted effort had been made to vary the appearance of the rooms.

In the total score calculated for environmental diversity there was a wide range (15 per cent – 59 per cent) between homes. Between voluntary and local authority homes there was a statistically significant difference in the mean scores, with greater diversity noted in the former group (mean scores 45.5 per cent and 35 per cent respectively; t = 2.32, p = 0.034). It will be recalled that a number of the voluntary homes were being extensively refurbished during the fieldwork period.

- *resident functioning — residents' appearance, amount of activity, interaction and verbal exchanges between residents*

In ten homes residents seen in public areas were considered to be very well groomed. Only in three homes was residents' clothing described as 'somewhat worn' or 'soiled'. Residents in most of the homes (28) were generally inactive and rarely seen to interact (27 homes). There was a wide range between homes in the total score for resident functioning (13.33 per cent to 73.3 per cent) and a significant difference between nursing and residential home mean scores, with lower levels of functioning in the former (mean scores 39.4 per cent and 56.6 per cent respectively; t = 3.275, p = 0.003).

- *staff functioning — quality of interaction and physical contact with residents, availability of staff to residents, organisation, staff conflict*

In general staff were considered to have a warm, if not personal manner when interacting with residents (27 homes). Fairly regular physical contact between staff and residents was also noted, at least to a moderate degree in 28 homes. Staff were usually accessible to residents in 19 homes, but in ten they were only available sometimes, or would have to be sought by residents who needed them. The researchers' ratings of the level of organisation in study homes were based on assessment of managerial organisation — for example clarity of staff roles and ability to access information; and of the provision of nursing and personal care to residents — whether care needs were seen to receive prompt and efficient attention. All but four of the homes were considered at least to be fairly well organised. The Rating Scale requires researchers to be aware of any subtle signs of friction, based on the expectation that staff may minimise conflict in public. 'Considerable' or 'moderate' conflict was observed in only two homes.

Rating the homes' environmental quality: researchers' general ratings

For this study, one general rating was added at the end of the MEAP Rating Scale, using terminology similar to that of a question included on the Relatives' Questionnaire. This invited researchers to consider each home in terms of how happy they would be to have a close relative living there. These overall ratings were compared to the four Rating Scale sub-scales. Between homes in which researchers would have been 'not happy', 'fairly happy' or 'very happy' to see a close relative there was little or no difference in the sub-scale ratings of physical attractiveness or diversity. A somewhat bigger difference between the three groups in staff functioning failed to reach statistical significance (Kruskall-Wallis test). Only in resident functioning was there a significant difference both between the 'not happy' and 'fairly happy' group (Mann-Whitney, $p = 0.001$) and between 'fairly happy' and 'very happy' ($p = 0.002$). It appears, therefore, that the researchers based their overall judgement of home quality on observation of residents, and possibly, though to a lesser extent, on staff. The physical environment was a much less significant feature of this judgement.

Rating the homes' environmental quality: researchers' and relatives' ratings compared

Use of this one general rating question by both researchers and relatives permits comparison between the two. It is noteworthy that there was no relationship between the researchers' and the relatives' ratings of the study homes ($r = 0.287$).

The residents

During the 15-month recruitment period 472 referrals were received from the original 35 homes. Of these, 70 were excluded before admission to the study, because they died or moved out before interview, were referred too late to be seen within the 14-day limit or turned out to be short-term or respite care admissions. The 36 who were referred too late represent a small percentage of the total but do illustrate the difficulty of ensuring that referrals are made within a tight deadline. This number would probably have been higher without the project team's practice of making regular telephone calls to the homes.

Of the remaining 402 eligible residents, ten residents had to be excluded when five homes were withdrawn due to their inability to provide sufficient referrals to the study. A further 84 residents refused to participate. A small number of refusals were given by the home, or by a relative on behalf of a resident prior to any direct contact but the majority came from residents themselves. A few residents withdrew consent during interview and were removed from the study. Thus the study's refusal rate was 20.9 per cent. In one of the few available comparisons, Bury and Holme (1990) reported a refusal rate of 17.6 per cent from a sample of people aged over 90 living in their own homes or in residential care. By this standard a refusal rate of 20.9 per cent with people very recently subjected to the upheaval of moving to a care home seems reasonable.

There is very little information available about the refusers, since once a refusal was made it was inappropriate to press the resident for detailed explanation or to gather further information from the home. There are no data available about their mental state or physical condition on admission so it is not possible to compare refusers with the final cohort with regard to cognitive impairment or dependency level. However, refusers and participants did not differ significantly in age group or whether they were in nursing or residential homes. From what residents said to the researchers when refusing it appears that they had a variety of reasons which would not suggest that they were concentrated in more or less disabled groups. On the one hand some residents who appeared very active said they had no time and politely made it plain that they had better things to do. On the other hand there were residents who felt too ill and weak to be bothered with research questions. Some residents were particularly apprehensive about being asked memory questions. These were people who were experiencing problems and had perhaps been recently tested in hospital. It seems likely that some of these residents refused because they did not want their problem further exposed, to themselves or to others.

In total 308 residents were interviewed in the 30 homes of the final study sample, comprising 65.3 per cent of the total residents originally referred. Most came from the Cheshire (48 per cent) and Blackpool (38 per cent) areas, with only 14 per cent from Manchester. They were evenly divided between nursing and residential homes, with 51.6 per cent (n=159) being nursing home residents. The largest proportion of residents was in private homes (44.5 per cent), followed by voluntary homes (38.6 per cent), and the smallest number were in local authority homes (n=52, 16.9 per cent). It should be remembered that the voluntary homes included a number of former local authority homes transferred to independent control.

Immediately prior to admission, 44 per cent of residents were in hospital with 30 per cent coming directly from their own homes and the remainder admitted from relatives' homes and other nursing and residential homes. They were predominantly female (69 per cent) and white (all but two of the 308). Their ages ranged from 65 to 101 years, with a mean age of 83 (std.dev. 7.6 years). There were no significant differences in mean age between the three geographical areas or between nursing and residential home residents. Twenty-five per cent of the cohort was aged 90 years and over on admission.

It was only possible to collect data on marital status and number of children from residents who had sufficient memory to be eligible for the quality of life interview. Of the cohort of 308, 199 residents gave their marital status. Only 9 per cent had never been married and 18 per cent were still married, although not necessarily living with their spouse. The mean number of children was

1.62, although 28 per cent of the 199 had never had children. Government statistics (HMSO, 1975) indicate that for marriages between 1920 and 1939 the mean number of children per household ranged from 2.38 (1920–1924) to 2.03 (1935–1939), suggesting that these residents had below average family sizes. Peace et al., (1979) found that 41 per cent of the residential home residents interviewed had never had children. The 28 per cent in this study seems much lower than this, although still indicating over-representation of childless people in care home admissions. It is tempting to speculate that in 1979 childlessness may have been a somewhat stronger determinant of institutional admission than it is now, possibly because the increased age and disability of new admissions in the late 1990s was such as to make family support factors relatively less significant.

A limited approach was taken to social classification because it rapidly became apparent that the detailed questioning necessary to discriminate between various levels of 'white collar' employment did not produce reliable results. The study included a large number of women who described themselves as having been housewives. Further questioning about husbands' occupations often proved to be problematic, with many residents unclear about the precise nature of their (usually late) husbands' employment, which may have ceased 20–30 years previously. If they ever knew the exact job title or the number of employees or subordinates for whom their husbands were responsible this had long since been forgotten.

It was therefore decided to classify residents into two groups using the National Readership Survey ABCDE classification (Monk, 1985), but collapsing categories so that occupational groups A, B and C1 were combined, as were groups C2, D and E. This has the effect of dividing people into two (manual and non-manual) occupational groups. It should however be noted that the A/B/C1 category covers a very wide range of occupations from junior clerks to senior professionals and owners or managers of large public companies. Groups C2 and D include all skilled, semi-skilled or unskilled manual workers and the E classification is for people dependent on long-term state benefit. Because there was only one person in the E group this was combined with C2 and D. The almost complete absence of people from social class E may reflect the fact that, although some residents had experienced periods of unemployment, receipt of long-term state benefit is more common in subsequent generations. It is also less likely that people who spend most of their lives on state benefits because of unemployment or incapacity for work will survive to old age.

Social class data were collected on 193 residents who completed the LQOLP-R, which although it only represents just under two-thirds of the total cohort (62.7 per cent), does give some indication of the cohort's social class composition. Just over one-third were in group A/B/C1, representing a range of professional and non-manual occupations, with the other two-thirds in the group C2/D/E.

Studies of social trends in the nineteenth and twentieth centuries indicate that women married to manual workers tend to have more children than women married to non-manual workers (Macfarlane and Mugford, 1984). The average number of children in manual / unskilled households ranged from 2.73 for marriages between 1920 and 24, to 2.49 for marriages between 1925 and 1929 (Pearce and Britton, 1977). These figures are rather higher than those quoted above for the population as a whole. Since two-thirds of this study's residents came from social class groups C2/D/E, this does support the interpretation that older people with no or few offspring are over-represented in long stay care facilities.

Because the study had been set in three very different areas of the north-west the list of former occupations of participants or their spouses reflected the social history of this part of the world. The largest town in the studied area of Cheshire was Crewe, and occupations included railway workers of various kinds described in terms used in the age of steam: footplateman or fireman. There were also agricultural labourers, farmers and the occasional landowner who strongly objected to being described as a farmer. In Manchester many of the women had been employed outside the home, often in the cotton industry; there were also academics, engineers and people who had worked at senior level in public corporations. In the Blackpool area the study encountered many people who had, during working life, lived in Manchester or the surrounding industrial towns. Occasionally a retired cotton spinner or weaver would demonstrate the art of 'mee-mawing'.[1] People who had been employed in the hotel and catering industries of the area were also represented, as were trawler fishermen from Fleetwood.

At the end of the fieldwork period, homes were asked, in relation to each study resident, whether care in the home had been paid for privately or with partial or full use of public funds. This information was only available for 215 residents (including 120 of the 159 in nursing homes). This was because some homes did not have the information, sometimes as a matter of deliberate policy, and others refused to divulge it. This means that the data must be used with care, because of the possibility of systematic bias. For example, the information was unavailable for a significantly greater proportion of residential home (37 per cent) than nursing home (24 per cent) residents. With that caution, it can be reported that, of the 215 residents for whom information was available, one-third paid for their care entirely from their own resources. When this is related to social class the combined effect of 'missing values' for both pieces of information means that the numbers, unfortunately, become even smaller. Based on the 132 residents for whom both social class and

---

1   Exaggerated lip movements used to aid lip reading in Lancashire cotton mills.

payment status were known, 60 per cent of those who paid for their own care in full were in the non-manual social classes A/B/C1.

Residents' daily lives: the observation study

Methods

In general, the methods used for collecting information about the care environment were those of staff interview and questionnaire. The study's ability to characterise aspects of this environment was, however, enriched by the addition of two methods of enquiry which were based on direct observation, the MEAP environmental rating scale, described above, and the observation study which is the subject of this section. For this, a structured method of non-participant observation was developed for the study, as described in Chapter 3 and Appendix 1, based on a time sampling technique similar to that used by Lemke and Moos (1984). Researchers conducted a 'sweep' of the home at set time periods between 10 a.m. and 5 p.m., recording the location, activity and verbal or physical 'contacts' of all residents visible in public space. Full details of the observation categories appear in Appendix 1 but are summarised below to assist interpretation of what follows.

Private / public space The number of occupied beds in the home was recorded before each observation session. Each resident in public space' was observed, that is, everyone who could be seen in hallways, lounges, dining rooms or gardens. Residents who were in bedrooms or bathrooms were in 'private space' and were not observed. The proportion of residents in public space was calculated in relation to the total occupied beds on that day.

Activities The main activity categories recorded for residents in public space were:
  Sleeping/dozing This was used when the resident appeared to be asleep, with eyes shut. Used conservatively by researchers, this category describes a situation in which there was no other observable behaviour, for example the activity of a dozing resident being pushed in a wheelchair would have been recorded as 'locomotion'.
  Awake The resident's eyes were open but there was no other observable behaviour.
  Group activities Social or recreational activities such as card games or exercises involving more than one resident, visitor or staff member.
  Individual activities Several individual activities were recorded, including 'individual pursuits' (such as knitting, sewing, reading), 'watching TV or listening to the radio' (used only when the resident appeared to be paying

attention to the broadcast), 'chores' (setting tables, making drinks, dusting) and 'self care' (combing hair, applying make-up).

Eating / drinking The resident was either actively doing this or sitting at a set table waiting for a meal.

Locomotion Any form of resident movement (including being wheeled or transferred).

Staff–resident contact Any verbal and /or physical contact between residents and home staff or visiting professionals was recorded. Contact with up to two members of staff could be recorded at one observation.

Verbal activity Residents' verbal activities were recorded under the following main categories: silent; loud speech (including shouting or arguing); quiet speech (not directed or conversational); noise (repetitive or incomprehensible utterances; screaming); 'being spoken to' (one way verbal contact, with the resident on the receiving end) and conversation.

Before considering what this exercise produced, some points should be noted about the data and how these were used to create some summary variables. First, it must be emphasised that the method involved time sampling rather than continuous observation and thus produced snapshots of behaviour. This means that the data cannot provide a measure of the duration of any activity or contact. Second, as with all time sampling methods there are limits to the claims which can be made for its representativeness. To substantiate a claim to represent the total experience of residents in a home would involve doing a sufficiently large, and randomly distributed, number of observations to represent an unknowable (but, in terms of the data collection task, very long) period of time. No such claim is made here. However, despite its inevitable limitations in this respect, the observation study was designed to produce a large number of observations on different days in different homes and done according to a consistent procedure. It is considered that this provides a reasonable picture of particular aspects of daily life within the study homes.

When compared with observation methods which use continuous recording techniques, time sampling tends to under-estimate behaviours which are of short duration. More confidence can, therefore, be placed in this study's findings on long duration behaviours or states such as sitting or sleeping than in findings on short duration behaviours such as brief verbal exchanges.

In order to standardise the data, aggregated variables were created so that all the observed categories are expressed in relation to the number of occupied beds. For example, a statement that 'x per cent of home y's residents were in public space at 11 a.m.' would mean that the number of residents observed in public space at that time had been divided by the number of occupied beds on that day and multiplied by 100. Descriptive statistics for the activities and contacts are presented and tested in various ways but all are based on this procedure. Where means are given, unless otherwise specified, these are means across all homes and all time periods. Summary variables were created to differentiate between residents who were, in general terms, occupied or unoccupied, grouping in various ways observations where the resident was sitting in silence, awake or dozing and not engaged in any other observable behaviour.

Findings

The extent to which residents' daily lives were spent predominantly in 'public' or 'private' space was one of the main environmental characteristics the observation study was designed to investigate. It must be emphasised that this was regarded as lifestyle indicator without making any judgement about whether one is better than the other. Whether residents who spent most of their time alone in their own rooms were happier or better off than those who were usually in the company of others was not a question for the observation study. It was designed simply to record the difference.

Across all homes and all observation times, on average 63 per cent of residents were visible, that is in 'public space', but the range was considerable (std.dev. 19 per cent, min. 9.68 per cent, max. 100 per cent). In general, variation did not occur in relation to the time of day except when mealtimes were compared with other times as a specific category. When all times were compared using one-way ANOVA there were no significant differences in the proportion of residents in public space between times. However, using a t-test to compare mealtimes (12 noon, 1 p.m. and 5 p.m.) as a group with all other times, the difference was highly significant (t = –3.43, p = 0.001). Thus, in homes where residents spent a high proportion of time in private, it appears that they emerged only for meals. It was also possible that nursing homes might have differed from residential homes in this respect, for example because nursing home residents might be more likely to be bed bound due to physical impairment. However, there was no significant difference between nursing and residential homes in the proportion of residents in 'public space' (t-test).

Figure 4.1 illustrates, across all homes and all times, the proportion of residents engaged in various activities (or inactivities). On average 23 per cent of the homes' residents were in public space and sitting, but not engaged in any other activity. A further 10 per cent were sleeping or dozing in public space. Altogether 9.8 per cent were engaged in individual (8.4 per cent) or group (1.4 per cent) activities.

There were significant differences at different times of the day. Predictably the majority of residents were eating and drinking at the 12 noon, 1 p.m. and 5 p.m. observation rounds. At 5 p.m. residents were less likely to be asleep or sitting doing nothing. while group activities were relatively rare, when they were observed this was most likely to be between 3 p.m. and 4 p.m. Examining all forms of individual and group activity there was a significant difference across time periods (one-way ANOVA p = 0.002).

Figure 4.1
Observed resident activities

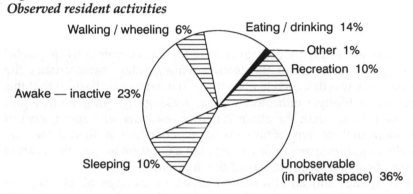

Note: 30 homes, all observations.

Although nursing home residents might have been expected to be less likely to engage in activities because of physical disability the proportion of residents who were either awake and doing nothing or asleep did not differ significantly between nursing and residential homes (t-test). However, residents in residential homes were more likely to be moving about (t = 2.83, p = 0.09), involved in individual pursuits (t = –3.58, p = 0.001), watching TV or listening to the radio (t = 2.64, p = 0.014).

Staff contact with residents, either verbal or physical, was rarely observed. On average only 6 per cent of residents were in public space and in contact with staff (std.dev. 2.8 per cent, min. 1.2 per cent, max. 12.9 per cent). There were no significant differences between different times of day, or between nursing and residential homes. Table 4.6 shows residents' verbal and physical contacts with qualified nurses, other care staff or visiting professionals. On average only 1 per cent of residents were in any kind of contact with qualified nurses and 4.4 per cent with other care staff.

Figure 4.2 shows that on average almost half the residents were observed to be silent. Only 13.7 per cent of residents were observed in any kind of verbal activity, including 9.5 per cent in conversation. Residents in private space may, of course, have been involved in verbal activity, perhaps retiring to their own

Table 4.6
Verbal and physical contacts with nurses, care staff or visiting professionals

	Mean	Std dev.	Min.	Max.
% of residents in contact with nurse	0.95	1.11	0	4.34
% of residents in contact with other care staff	4.42	2.4	1.21	11.33
% of residents in contact with visiting professional	0.41	1.01	0	5.3

Note: 30 homes, all observations.

rooms when they had company. Significant differences in residents' verbal interactions were associated with mealtimes. When grouped mealtimes (12 noon, 1 p.m. and 5 p.m.) were compared with all other times residents were more likely to be silent or being spoken to at mealtimes, ($t = -2.51, p = 0.0135$ and $t = -2.87, p = 0.004$ respectively).

It might have been expected that nursing home residents would be less likely to participate in conversation because of greater cognitive impairment. That there was greater cognitive impairment in the nursing homes was supported by the study's interviews with residents (to be reported in Chapter 5). There was indeed less conversation observed in the nursing homes. On average 11.1 per cent of residential home residents and 6.5 per cent of nursing home residents were observed in conversation ($t = 3.39, p = 0.002$).

Figure 4.2
Observed verbal contacts

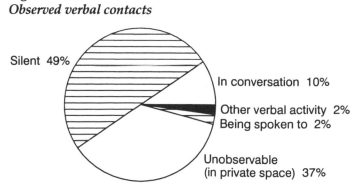

In summary

- A large proportion of private homes and local authority homes were represented in the study sample. Staff / resident ratio was highest in nursing homes but there was considerable variation within each staff group.

- Care assistant time per occupied bed in residential homes ranged from half an hour to two and three-quarter hours a day, and in nursing homes from two and a half hours to five hours per day. Few homes had qualified or unqualified 'activity' or therapy staff and 80 per cent provided less than six minutes 'activity' per day.
- There was great variation in charges and a small number of homes charged extra for services such as chiropody or physiotherapy.
- The MEAP rating of home environmental quality found that most homes were rated as attractive and reasonably well-maintained, free from unpleasant odours and reasonably clean in public living areas. There was evidence of variation and personalisation of most residents' rooms. However, the homes in which researchers felt happy to place a relative of their own were those rated better for resident functioning rather than physical environment.
- The observation study revealed little evidence of residents engaged in activities in either nursing or residential homes. There was little evidence of contact, either physical or verbal between staff and residents. Residents observed in public space were rarely seen to be in conversation with other residents or staff.

5 Residents' Health and Quality of Life

This chapter examines the mental health, physical health and aspects of quality of life in residents soon after their admissions to residential or nursing care homes.

Psychiatric morbidity

Psychiatric disorders in residents, both organic and functional, were a major focus of the study, and the screening assessment carried out in the first phase of interviewing provides an estimate of their prevalence in new admissions to homes during this period (Mozley et al., 2000). Most of the epidemiological studies referred to in Chapter 2 were cross-sectional, involving all, or a sample of all, home residents. The disadvantage of this approach is that the condition of residents on entry is disguised, on the one hand, by the effects of improvement due to factors such as improved diet and, on the other hand, by deterioration of frail residents over time. New admission studies aid, amongst other things, consideration of the requirements for pre-admission assessment.

As described in Chapter 3, the primary method used for assessing cognitive impairment in the residents was the Mini Mental State Examination, or MMSE. Of the 308 residents, it was impossible to complete the MMSE with 14 people who were completely unresponsive or unwilling to proceed. The mean score of 14 for the remainder indicates a considerable degree of cognitive impairment. Figure 5.1 shows the percentage within each cognitive impairment category, using the three cut-points described by Tombaugh and McIntyre (1992), with the additional cut-point of 9/10 used in this study to provide a more conservative definition of severity as a screen for further, quality of life

Figure 5.1
MMSE scores

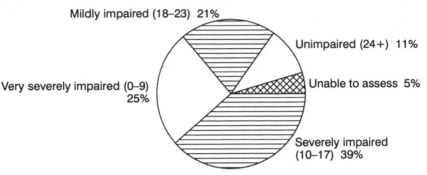

Mildly impaired (18–23) 21%

Unimpaired (24+) 11%

Very severely impaired (0–9)
25%

Unable to assess 5%

Severely impaired
(10–17) 39%

interviewing. Using the 17/18 MMSE cut-point to demarcate severe cognitive impairment means that almost two-thirds could be considered severely impaired. Even if the term 'severe' is regarded as a little extreme for all scores below 18, it seems clear that in a high proportion of those interviewed marked impairment was present. Only 11 per cent of respondents scored 24 or more (out of 30) and could be considered unimpaired.

The MMSE was supplemented by the Abbreviated Mental Test Score, or AMTS. These two measures of cognitive impairment were strongly correlated ($r = 0.847$, $p < 0.001$). With the commonly used MMSE and AMTS cut-points only 36 (12.2 per cent) of the 294 'measurable' residents had scores for the two measures which disagreed as to the presence of cognitive impairment. Of these, two-thirds were mildly impaired according to the MMSE (18–23) and unimpaired according to the AMTS.

MMSE score was not significantly correlated with age; nor were any score differences associated with gender or geographical area. There was, however, an association with social class. Based on the 193 residents for whom social class data were available, median MMSE scores were 21 and 16 for residents in classes A/B/C1 and C2/D respectively (Mann-Whitney $U = 3085.5$, $p = 0.001$), indicating a higher proportion of cognitively impaired residents in the lower social class. This difference may, in part, be one of test performance rather than of underlying impairment — O'Connor et al. (1989) found that MMSE scores are affected by education and social class — but it seems unlikely that this would account fully for so large a difference. Of the 215 residents for whom information was available on who paid for their care, those who paid entirely from private funds were less cognitively impaired, with a median MMSE score of 17.5 compared with 12 for those who were publicly funded (Mann-Whitney $U = 2936.5$, $p < 0.001$).

Residents who had come to the home direct from hospital were more impaired than those who had not, with median MMSE scores for the two groups of 13 and 15 respectively (Mann-Whitney U = 9205, p = 0.056). As might be expected, new admissions to nursing homes were more impaired. Median MMSE scores were 12 and 16 respectively in the nursing and residential home residents (Mann-Whitney U = 8062.5, p <0.001). However, if the 17/18 cut-point is used, although the nursing and residential home groups differed significantly in the proportion of severely impaired new admissions (χ^2 (1) = 5.55, p = 0.018) as many as 61 per cent of new admissions in residential homes came into this category.

Cognitive impairment and dependency were closely linked, as demonstrated by statistically significant correlations between MMSE and both Barthel and Crichton Royal scores. The latter was more strongly correlated with the MMSE (r = –0.606, p < 0.001) than was the Barthel (r = 0.369, p < 0.001) because it contains items on memory, orientation and communication while the Barthel concentrates more exclusively on the physical manifestations of dependency.

The Crichton Royal, included in the informant interviews, provided a staff rating of the resident's orientation to place. This was used to investigate the extent to which staff assessments agreed with MMSE findings. One of the seven MMSE domains tests orientation to place, with a maximum of 5 points being available for this. Residents who scored 3 or more were categorised as oriented to place. The Crichton Royal orientation ratings were categorised so that a rating of 2 or less (on a scale of 0: complete orientation, to 4: completely lost) indicated orientation. Of the 300 residents for whom both measures are available there was disagreement in 101 cases. However only 17 (12 per cent) of those who were oriented to place according to the MMSE were described by staff as disoriented. Thus staff were rarely likely to perceive cognitively intact residents as impaired although they were less clear in the reverse situation. Given that these were very recent admissions this suggests that staff were not willing to judge people as cognitively impaired on the basis of short acquaintance and little evidence.

Of the 308 residents, 46 (15 per cent) were unable fully to complete the Geriatric Depression Scale. Some of these were unresponsive or unwilling to complete the assessment; some failed to understand the questions. Scores were treated as missing where three or more items were unanswered. This left 248 residents with valid GDS-15 scores. These 248 residents had a mean GDS-15 score of 5.4 (std.dev. 3.2). Using the conventional cut-point of 5/6, just under 45 per cent were depressed 'cases'. Excluding residents with very low MMSE scores (below 10) does not alter this figure because all but 11 of the low MMSE scorers were in fact excluded by the requirement that only two unanswered items were allowed. The shorter forms of the GDS-15 (GDS-4 and GDS-10) were derived from the responses obtained for the 15-item scale with 'caseness' cut-points of 0/1 for the former and 2/3 for the latter, as recommended by Shah et al. (1997). Both gave much higher 'caseness' rates — 67.3 per cent for the ten-item and 55.6 per cent for the four-item version, compared with 44.8 per cent for the full scale.

There was no statistically significant difference in depression 'caseness' between the groups in nursing and residential homes. The GDS-15 was not significantly correlated with the MMSE. There were no significant associations between depression and age, gender, or care home sector but there was an association with social class. Of the 185 residents for whom both valid GDS-15 scores and social class data were available 48 per cent overall were depressed. However 39 per cent of those in classes A/B/C1 were depressed, compared with 54 per cent of those in C2/D $(\chi^2(1) = 4.10, p = 0.043)$.

Depression was correlated with both dependency measures used in the study, in the expected direction — higher GDS-15 scores being correlated with greater dependency, although in both cases the values were low (GDS-15/Barthel r = –0.240, p < 0.001; GDS-15/Crichton Royal r = 0.166, p = 0.009). Additionally, there was a significant difference between depressed and non-depressed residents in their own ratings, on a five-point scale, of current general health status (Mann-Whitney U = 4449, p < 0.001).

The depression scores were also examined in relation to some specific disabilities. There was no association between depression and incontinence. There was a statistically significant association with reduced mobility as measured both by the Barthel (Mann-Whitney U = 6546, p = 0.04) and the Crichton Royal (Mann-Whitney U = 5855, p = 0.002). Depression 'caseness' was not associated with hearing loss but it was associated with visual impairment $(\chi^2(1) = 4.335, p = 0.037)$. It should be noted here that some caution is required in interpreting the data on sensory impairment because they were not derived from direct assessment and staff were often somewhat uncertain about these matters.

Thus it seems clear that older people now being admitted to care homes include a high proportion of those with clinically significant cognitive impairment; and that this is closely related to high dependency in daily living activities. The study also supports other research findings (Mann et al., 1984; Ames et al., 1988; Schneider et al., 1997a) that depression is present in very high proportions of care home residents. Of this study's cohort of residents assessed shortly after admission only 10 per cent were free from cognitive impairment, compared with 21 per cent in the residential home sample studied in 1994–1996 by Schneider et al. (1997a,b,c); and the depression 'caseness' prevalence of 45 per cent was somewhat higher. Some caution must be exercised in interpreting these comparisons because different measurement instruments were used. Moreover, MMSE scores may be lowered to some extent by the effects of recent admission, particularly on orientation, and the fact of recent admission may also be responsible for increased depression prevalence.

There was considerable evidence of co-morbidity of cognitive impairment and depression in this cohort of newly admitted residents. Of the 308, 61 per cent had at least one of these problems, suffering from severe cognitive impairment (MMSE < 18) or depression (GDS-15 > 5) or both conditions concurrently. Co-morbidity of these two conditions was found in 24 per cent; it is impossible to know whether, in addition, some of the severely cognitively impaired residents for whom valid GDS-15 scores could not be computed were depressed.

Although cognitive impairment was significantly greater in nursing home admissions, severe impairment was present in 61 per cent of new admissions to the 18 residential homes, only one of which had special responsibility to care for the 'elderly mentally infirm'. The data collected from homes prior to the fieldwork period (see Chapter 4) provide information about the disabilities of the whole resident population of 1057 people living in the 30 homes before admission of the cohort members. The presence of short-term memory problems was identified in approximately two-thirds of both groups (66.4 per cent of the total population and 68.7 per cent of the cohort). Similarly, disorientation was reported in 61.7 per cent of the population and 64.7 per cent of the cohort. No summary measure of depression in the whole population was available. These 'whole population' figures included residents who had been in the homes for some time and who might be expected to have experienced cognitive deterioration since admission. It is possible that this provides support for the frequently heard observation of care providers that people, on admission, are more cognitively impaired than in previous years. However, it must be recalled that in the new admission cohort, staff tended to underestimate cognitive impairment compared with MMSE assessment. The staff ratings on which the 'whole population' figures are based may similarly underestimate impairment.

It is noteworthy that residents in the lower social class were more cognitively impaired and more depressed. Although some of the cognitive impairment difference is probably attributable to measurement error, due to education and social class bias, it is unlikely that this provides full explanation of a median MMSE score difference of 5 points. Although caution is required because of incompleteness in the data on social class and on whether residents paid for their own care (see Chapter 4) it does tend to support a speculative interpretation that those who are dependent on state support have more psychiatric morbidity on admission than those who are able, with the power of the purse, to make their own admission decisions.

Dependency and physical morbidity

Information about each resident's dependency needs was obtained by interviewing staff informants, using the Barthel and the Crichton Royal (Challis et al., 2000b). It should be recalled here (from Chapter 3, where these instruments are described) that, for the Barthel a higher score (maximum 20) corresponds to a lower level of dependency and the Crichton Royal is scored in the opposite direction, with a higher score (maximum 38) indicating a higher level of dependency. Scores for these two measures derived from the assessment made shortly after admission were, as might be expected, highly correlated ($r = -0.791$, $p < 0.001$). However, skills in the individual items such as bathing or dressing are rated in ways which are not directly comparable. The major benefits of the Crichton Royal are that it includes items which can be treated as a distinct Confusion Sub-scale and that it permits a more detailed evaluation of the assistance required with bathing. Only the bathing assessment of the Crichton Royal is used in the following discussion of dependency levels, with reliance otherwise placed on the Barthel.

For the whole cohort the mean Barthel score was 11.4 (std.dev. 5.5). If the cut-points used in other studies (Granger et al., 1979; Darton and Brown, 1997) are applied this mean score was within a range which would be categorised as low–medium dependency. Fifteen per cent ($n=45$) were 'high dependency' (score 0–4), 17 per cent ($n=52$) 'medium dependency' (score 5–8), 18 per cent ($n=56$) 'low/medium dependency' (score 9–12) and 50 per cent ($n=155$) 'low dependency' (score 13–20).

Table 5.1 shows the proportion of cohort residents with specific dependency needs. For each activity of daily living a high proportion of these newly admitted residents needed considerable help from others. For the four activities for which comparable data were collected from home managers, the second column of this table shows the dependency needs of the whole population of these homes. The Barthel was not used for collecting 'whole population' data but the four-point rating scheme used provides a reasonable basis for comparison (see Appendix 2). Although the 'whole population' figures included longer-term residents who might be expected to have experienced deterioration, the new admission cohort contained a higher proportion of dependent people in three of the four activities, and a similar proportion of dependency for incontinence of urine.

There was a statistically significant difference in the Barthel score between nursing and residential home residents, with means of 8.7 and 14.3 respectively (Mann-Whitney, $p < 0.001$), the nursing home residents being the more dependent. In Figures 5.2 and 5.3, residents in the two types of home are divided into dependency groups using the Barthel cut-points. Very few residential home residents had high dependency needs on admission, with 92

Table 5.1

Specific dependency needs of cohort members — some comparisons with whole population of study homes

	% of cohort with specific dependencies (n=308) ('Barthel' unless otherwise stated)	% of whole population of 30 homes with specific dependencies (n=1057)
Incontinent of faeces (regularly)	23	–
Incontinent of urine (regularly)	30	36
Need help to wash face/shave/do hair/clean teeth	55	42
Need some help to use WC (i.e. help on/off; wiping)	55	39
Need some help with feeding (at least food cutting etc.)	29	–
Need help of two people to transfer bed/chair	33	–
Have no mobility (cannot walk even with aids or help of one person; not independent using wheelchair)	24	–
Need at least some help to walk or wheel indoors	58	44
Need to be dressed (unable to do at least half the task unaided)	35	–
Unable to manage stairs*	83	–
Need major help with bathing (able, at best, to wash own hands and face with supervision) (Crichton Royal)	45	–

Note: * Responses to this item affected by home policy and building design.

per cent in the two lower dependency groups. In the cohort as a whole, Barthel and MMSE scores were significantly correlated (r = 0.340, p = 0.001) making it unlikely that admission of many of the lower dependency residents was due to severe cognitive impairment. Among the 105 residential home admissions in the lowest dependency group the mean MMSE was 16 (std.dev. 6.9).

In nursing homes, although there were far higher proportions of high dependency residents, as many as 31 per cent were in the low dependency group. The mean Barthel score for the 49 nursing home admissions in the low dependency group was 15.3 (std.dev. 1.9) and the mean MMSE score 15.2 (std.dev. 8). Of these 49 residents, 44 were independently mobile, 38 were fully continent and 36 went to the toilet and used it independently. Possible reasons for admission to the nursing homes of these low dependency people were investigated. Potential explanatory variables were identified and, using χ^2, t-tests and Mann Whitney U tests as appropriate, the low dependency group

Figure 5.2
Barthel dependency groups (residential homes)

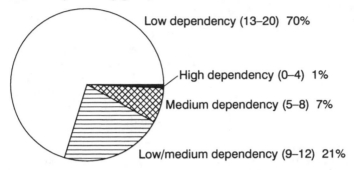

Figure 5.3
Barthel dependency groups (nursing homes)

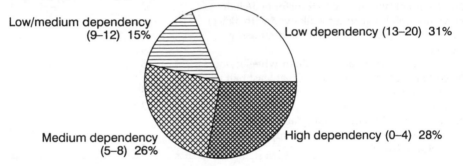

was compared with a group comprising all other nursing home residents. There were no statistically significant differences between these two groups in any of the areas shown in Table 5.2. The two groups were significantly different in MMSE scores, with the low dependency group, as might be expected, being less cognitively impaired ($t = -3.36$ (d.f. 144), $p = 0.001$). The only statistically significant difference which offered a possible explanation of the low dependency nursing home admissions was in whether or not residents were self-funding.

Information about payment was available for a total of 120 of the 159 nursing home admissions, the missing data resulting from the fact that some homes did not have this information available and others refused to divulge it. To check for any systematic bias Barthel scores were compared for the two groups. There was no statistically significant difference between the 'data available' (mean score 8.7) and 'data unavailable' (8.4) groups. Based on the data for the 120 residents, in the nursing homes low dependency was

Table 5.2
Nursing home admissions: low dependency versus others

No statistically significant between-group differences in:

- Age[a]
- Gender[b]
- Social class[b]
- Whether or not they were currently married[b]
- Whether or not they had children[b]
- Whether or not they had been admitted from hospital[b]
- Whether they were in homes in South Manchester, South Cheshire or Blackpool, Wyre and Fylde[b]
- The length of time taken by visiting relatives to get to the home[a]
- Whether relatives visited more or less often than weekly[b]
- Whether or not they had been diagnosed with a cardiovascular disorder[b]
- Whether or not they had been diagnosed with cancer (any kind)[b]
- Whether or not they had been diagnosed with a rheumatological disorder[b]
- Whether or not they had been diagnosed with dementia[b]
- Whether or not they had been diagnosed with a psychiatric disorder other than dementia[b]
- Whether or not they had been diagnosed with a respiratory disorder[b]
- Whether or not they had been diagnosed with diabetes[b]
- Whether or not they had been diagnosed with a neurological disorder[b]
- The number of diagnosed disorders (one counted for each of the above groupings)[c]
- Depression, measured by GDS-15[c]

Notes:
a. t-test.
b. χ^2 test.
c. Mann-Whitney U test.

significantly associated with paying for care exclusively from private resources ($\chi^2(1) = 9.00$, p = 0.003). Of those who are known to have paid in full for their own nursing home care, 67 per cent (31/46) were in the low dependency group. This situation was not observed in the residential homes.

Figure 5.4 shows the percentage of residential and nursing home residents with disorders in the most common (including at least ten residents) diagnostic groups, based on the information supplied to the home on admission. The most common diagnosis was of a non-stroke cardiovascular disorder (among the 308 there were 94 sufferers), followed by rheumatological diseases (62/308), dementia (58/308), stroke (57/308) and neurological disorders (39/308). With only one exception, there was no statistically significant association between type of home and having any of the grouped diagnoses shown. Exceptionally,

Figure 5.4
Common diagnoses in residential and nursing homes

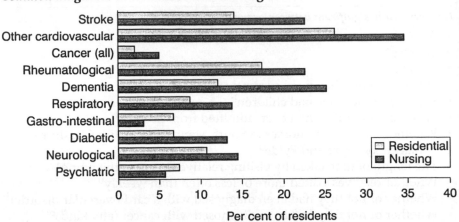

Per cent of residents

residents with a dementia diagnosis were more likely to be in nursing care ($\chi^2(1)$ = 8.61, p = 0.003).

Residents with a dementia diagnosis had significantly lower MMSE scores (mean 8.5) than those with no such diagnosis (mean score 15) (t = 6.595 (d.f. 292), p< 0.001) but the majority of low, or very low MMSE scorers had no dementia diagnosis. When the three diagnostic groupings of dementia, neurological disorder and 'other psychiatric' were aggregated, to include all likely explanations of cognitive impairment there was no significant association between MMSE score and diagnosis. Of 47 residents who scored 9 or less on the MMSE, indicating severe cognitive impairment, 40 (85 per cent) had no diagnosis in this aggregated category.

A number of the residents had one or more conditions which might be thought likely to benefit from active rehabilitation — for example 35 per cent of the residents suffered from rheumatological diseases and/or had had strokes. Although the extent to which any individual resident might have benefited from rehabilitation is not known, as described in Chapter 4, therapy or activity staff, qualified or unqualified, were rare in these 30 homes. Eighty per cent of the homes provided less than six minutes of 'activity staff' time per occupied bed per day; fourteen homes had none at all. No trained occupational therapists were employed. One home provided on-site physiotherapy services.

Figure 5.5 shows residents' prescribed medication, broken down according to British National Formulary classification. Central nervous system medication was the most common category, prescribed for 69 per cent of residents, followed by cardiovascular and gastro-intestinal drugs, prescribed for 62 per cent and 50 per cent respectively. The mean number of drugs per person was

Figure 5.5
Prescribed medication (BNF classification groups)

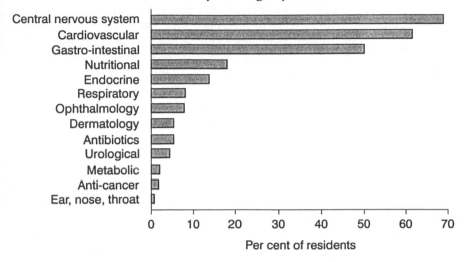

Per cent of residents

4.05 (std.dev. 2.75, range 0–13), with 52 per cent of residents on four or more drugs, the level at which adverse drug reactions become more common (Shaw and Opit, 1976). Furniss and colleagues (2000) found that 64 per cent of residents were prescribed four or more medications in a case-control intervention study of medication carried out with nursing home residents in Manchester. The mean numbers of drugs prescribed per resident were 5.1 and 4.9 for cases and controls respectively at baseline interview.

Previous studies have reported that residents suffering from more severe cognitive impairment are less likely to be prescribed analgesic medication (for example, Horgas and Tsai, 1998). Although a pain assessment was not included in this study it is worth noting that 46 per cent (n=87) of residents who scored 10 or more on the MMSE were prescribed analgesics, compared with only 26.4 per cent (n=23) of those who scored less than 10. This was a statistically significant difference (Mann-Whitney U, p = 0.014).

Psychiatric and physical morbidity — some policy observations

For many years a key feature of social policy has been to target residential resources upon the most dependent individuals, with a focus on home based care for those with lower dependency needs. It is, therefore, surprising to note that 71 per cent of new admissions to the residential homes and 31 per cent of new admissions to the nursing homes had low dependency needs. The only evidence of effective targeting would appear to be the fact that there were hardly any high dependency new admissions to the residential homes.

That this study found a significant proportion of new residential and nursing home admissions with low dependency needs is relevant to the question of whether greater diversion to home based care is feasible. At the time of this study, a residential care allowance of £50 per week was paid by the Department of Social Security to support publicly funded residents in private and voluntary homes. It was proposed in the White Paper *Modernising Social Services* (Cm 4169, 1998) that this be removed and the funding allocated to Social Services (para 7.25, 7.26). This was equivalent to raising the unit cost of residential or nursing home care by the amount of the residential care allowance. Such a relative price effect strengthens the case for home based care of people who are at the margin of needing institutional provision — since the opportunity cost of the allowance approximates to six hours of home care per week. There is some evidence that such marginal changes in the balance of care are possible at the local level (Challis and Hughes, 2002).

The need for appropriate assessment of older people prior to long-term care admission has been discussed in the literature for many years (Brocklehurst et al., 1978; Rafferty et al., 1987; Peet et al., 1994; Sharma et al., 1994). This is a topical issue in view of government concern about the need to improve multidisciplinary assessment procedures for vulnerable older people (Department of Health, 1997; Challis et al., 1998), exemplified in the establishment of the Single Assessment Process (Department of Health, 2002a). In this connection it was notable that nearly one-third of the new admissions to nursing home care had low dependency needs, and that these people were more likely to be self-funding. One explanation of this may be that those who are able to pay view nursing home care, with its medical associations, as less stigmatising than residential care, which may be seen as designed for those needing accommodation. These residents are attractive customers to nursing home operators faced with the challenge of low occupancy. It is also possible that relatives opt for nursing home care before it becomes necessary in order to avoid the distress of subsequent relocation.

It may appear that a choice of nursing home care taken by someone who is paying the full cost should not be a matter of concern for public policy. However, over a lengthy period in a nursing home private resources may be exhausted, leaving public authorities with a choice between moving the resident to a lower level of care elsewhere or continuing payment at the higher rate. Moreover, when low dependency people with financial resources opt for nursing home care they may be making a poor decision, inadequately informed by professional advice. They pay a higher price for a level of care they do not need, and may find themselves with fewer social opportunities because their fellow residents are more severely disabled, mentally and physically. For these reasons, the presence of significant numbers of low dependency residents in nursing homes suggests a need to provide better assessment and placement services for those who are financially independent of local authorities.

Because this study obtained MMSE scores for the cohort members, it was also possible to use these data to examine assessment practice in this particular area. Of those with MMSE scores of 9 or less, indicative of severe cognitive impairment, 85 per cent had no diagnosis of dementia, neurological disorder or any other psychiatric phenomena. This degree of apparent under-diagnosis of dementia is similar to that found by Iliffe et al. (1990) in a general practice study. Undoubtedly staff in the homes would, if asked, have described the majority of these people as suffering from dementia but they had been given no diagnosis. It should be added that some residential home staff commented that they were not given medical information as a matter of policy.

In general, the prevalence and degree of co-morbidity of cognitive impairment and depression in this sample raises questions, not only about the access of care home populations to specialist expertise in the diagnosis, treatment and management of these conditions, but also about the way in which critical placement decisions are made. The number of residents taking four or more drugs similarly raises questions about procedures for pre-admission medication review. The appropriate use of medicines for older people is highlighted in the *National Service Framework for Older People* (NSFOP) (Department of Health, 2001b). For older people, being prescribed four or more medicines has been identified as a risk factor for adverse drug reactions or for readmission to hospital. Furthermore, the study by Furniss and colleagues (2000) demonstrated that reducing the number of medicines prescribed for older people has no adverse effect on morbidity or mortality. The NSFOP *Medicines and Older People* (Department of Health, 2001c) has recommended that appropriate medicines management systems should be implemented in order to review the medication needs of older people. It has advised that care staff in residential homes require basic training on medicines, and an awareness of the potential for medication problems and what action needs to be taken, if necessary. Indeed, the effects of polypharmacy, particularly on balance, alertness or concentration can be such as to increase dependency. Unless this is taken into account before admission, inappropriate placement decisions may be made which are subsequently very difficult to reverse.

Residents' quality of life

A central theme of this study was residents' quality of life and how, if at all, this related to the quality of care provided. There is some controversy about the capacity of older people, particularly those suffering from cognitive impairment, to undertake a quality of life assessment (Albert, 1998). However, as described below, and more fully in Chapter 9, a high proportion of residents interviewed for this study were found to be capable of expressing a fairly reliable opinion about their life circumstances. In this chapter the results of 214 quality of life interviews with residents are reported. Of these, 213 scored 10 or more on the MMSE. The additional interviewee had stroke-related communication problems which made it impossible to answer MMSE questions, but most of the quality of life questions could be answered using gestures or pointing to the Likert scale show card.

The Lancashire Quality of Life Profile (Oliver et al., 1996) was, as described in Chapter 3, adapted for the particular needs of this study. Interpretation of the data produced by these interviews requires some preliminary remarks about these changes and the method used for score computation.

The original LQOLP includes a number of different sub-scales and global measures. Apart from the global ratings, they fall into one of the major life-domains. Each domain is made up of some objective ratings (such as the frequency of contact with relatives) and subjective ratings by the interviewee on a seven-point scale (known as the Life Satisfaction Scale or LSS). Because a five-point scale was found to be more readily understood by older people a change was made from practice with the original LQOLP. This must be taken into account when comparing the results of the present study with others where the longer scale has been used. The version used in this study compared with the original as follows:

General well-being

This single question counts as part of the total Life Satisfaction Scale (LSS): 'Can you tell me how you feel about your life as a whole today?' This was retained unaltered in the residential version.

Work/education

In the original, this section included three LSS questions with some additional non-LSS items. The whole section was omitted as irrelevant to older people in care homes.

Leisure/participation

This section was retained, including three LSS questions which ask the interviewee to rate pleasure derived from different types of activity.

Finance

The two LSS questions about money were retained.

Living situation

The six core questions of the original LSS sub-scale were retained (omitting only the optional question about possible return to hospital). To these were added six items covering:

- opportunities for going out;
- opportunities for keeping occupied;
- quality and variety of food;
- facilities for making own drinks / snacks;
- timing of breakfast; and
- ability to bring own possessions into the home.

Religion

Two questions about religious practice were included for an LSS sub-scale, as with the original, but instead of asking about satisfaction with 'your religious faith and its teachings', residents were asked about satisfaction with how often they were able to see a priest or minister.

Legal and safety

This LSS sub-scale was omitted as inapplicable in a residential situation. Residents were asked about safety and security in the home, but not in the LSS format.

Family relations

Instead of the three sub-scale items of the original LQOLP, residents were asked one question about satisfaction with the contact they had with relatives.

Social relations

The two LSS sub-scale items from the original were retained.

Health

The three sub-scale items of the original were retained, with one minor wording change, from 'how satisfied are you with your nervous well-being' to 'with the state of your nerves'.

Self concept

The ten self-concept scale items were converted into yes/no questions because the original was shown in piloting to be too complex for use with the study's interviewees.

Satisfaction with life as a whole

The one LSS item of the original was retained unaltered.

Cantril's ladder

This was retained, with simplified wording which did not require residents to think back to the life outcomes they might have expected.

   While interviewing residents it became apparent that many of them were reluctant to complain or criticise their care. In consequence it is believed that scores for sub-scales like living situation may be somewhat generous. It is not clear that this observation justifies making scoring adjustments. It is not the business of researchers to second-guess respondents — arguably, if they are not prepared to accept the answers given they should not ask questions. However, it was often the case that, given a five-point scale to choose from, residents would make it clear that they were using the mid point ('mixed / uncertain') as a way of expressing dissatisfaction — 'I shouldn't say I'm dissatisfied; you'd better put mixed/uncertain'. For this reason, it was decided to look at the scores in two ways. In addition to analysis of the global and sub-scale continuous scores, these have also been collapsed into binary variables which group 'very dissatisfied', 'mostly dissatisfied' and 'mixed / uncertain' into one 'dissatisfied' response, while 'mostly satisfied' and 'very satisfied' become one 'satisfied' response.
   Because it was anticipated that cognitive impairment would make it impossible to do quality of life interviewing with some residents, with only one exception, described above, the attempt was made only with those who scored 10 or more on the MMSE (see further Chapters 3 and 9). In all, 214 people were interviewed. Their mean age was 83.4 years (std.dev. 7.6 years), the youngest being 65 and the oldest 101. It is worth noting that one-quarter was aged 90 or over. The age distribution is different from that of the main cohort of 308. Only 30.4 per cent of the LQOLP-R interviewees were aged 79 or under, compared with 62 per cent of the whole cohort. Of the LQOLP-R interviewees, 72.4 per cent were female, and 55.6 per cent were in nursing homes.
   The existence of a relationship between quality of life and mood has been well established in research on people under 65 (Huxley, 1998). That there should be some relationship between depression and the perception of life

quality seems likely, but it is difficult to be clear about the direction of that relationship. Depressed mood may make respondents view the world in a worse light and thus give low quality or satisfaction ratings. Conversely life circumstances which offer few areas of satisfaction may result in depressed mood. People under 65 who have depressive symptoms remain able to discriminate between life domains in terms of their satisfaction, and in many samples even a diagnosis of depression does not lead to reduced subjective ratings in certain life domains (Huxley, 1998). In Figure 5.6 the depressed and non-depressed groups are compared.

Figure 5.6
Life satisfaction in depressed and non-depressed residents

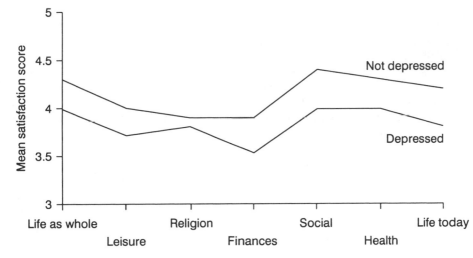

Of the 214 LQOLP-R interviewees, 45.6 per cent were depressed 'cases' using the 5/6 cut on the GDS-15. It can be seen that although the depressed people had consistently lower satisfaction ratings the pattern of responses on the different domains was similar. The depressed residents were still able to discriminate between different areas of life and were not overwhelmed in their judgement by their mood state.

The total LSS score and Cantril's ladder are measures of overall or global well-being. The LSS total score was significantly correlated with all the sub-scales and with Cantril's ladder (in all cases p <0.001). Cantril's ladder was significantly correlated (at the 0.01 level or better) with all the sub-scales except religion and social relations. It might be expected that residents' perceptions of their quality of life would be greatly affected by mental or physical disability. The correlation table displayed as Table 5.3 shows the relationship between

LSS total score, Cantril's ladder, cognitive impairment (MMSE), physical dependency (Barthel) and depression (GDS-15).

The LSS total score is significantly correlated (at the 0.01 level or better) with: Cantril's ladder (in the expected direction); the MMSE score (lower cognitive impairment being correlated with higher satisfaction); and the Barthel score (lower dependency correlated with higher satisfaction) and GDS-15 score (higher satisfaction correlated with a lower number of depressed responses). Therefore residents rating themselves as more satisfied with their lives were also more likely to: have better expectations of their lives (Cantril); be less cognitively impaired (MMSE); be rated as less dependent by staff (Barthel); rate themselves as less depressed (GDS-15) and be rated as having a better quality of life by the researchers (Uniscale). There were no statistically significant relationships between LSS total score and age or gender or with residence in nursing or residential sectors. LSS total scores were somewhat higher (greater satisfaction) among residents in the higher social class (Mann-Whitney, $p = 0.04$).

As part of the LSS the interviewed residents were asked to rate their satisfaction with life as a whole, and with life today (the two questions being separated by almost the whole interview). As Figures 5.7 and 5.8 show, the responses to the two questions indicate that a number of people were less satisfied with their present circumstances.

The mean scores for life as a whole and life today were 4.1 (std.dev. 0.8) and 3.75 (std.dev. 1.1) respectively, a difference which is statistically significant (paired samples $t = 4.42$, $p < 0.001$). It is hard to know how to interpret the difference. On the one hand, the difference may simply be due to the wording of the questions. Residents may be happier with life as a whole, and at the same time less happy about things on that particular day. On the other hand, the influence of responding to many questions about their life in the home may have had a downward influence on their ratings. This phenomenon has been observed in younger samples (Oliver et al., 1996), but tends to occur mostly in people who are already depressed at the start of the interview. Similarly, when one compares the depressed and non-depressed groups in the present sample one finds that the reduction in the ratings occurs almost exclusively in the depressed group, from a mean of 3.9 (std.dev. 0.9) to 3.3 (std.dev. 1.2), compared to a reduction for the non-depressed group from a mean of 4.3 (std.dev. 0.6) to 4.2 (std.dev. 0.8). This confirms the findings with younger samples and suggests that screening for depression should always accompany quality of life assessment. Having said that, the residents who were depressed were as satisfied with the home in general (mean 4.6) as those who were not (mean 4.7).

Also shown in Table 5.3 are the correlations with the Spitzer Uniscale completed by researchers, included to provide an independent assessment of the residents' quality of life. This is significantly correlated (at the 0.001 level)

Table 5.3
Life satisfaction scale, Cantril's Ladder, MMSE, Barthel and GDS-15 Scores and Spitzer Uniscale: correlations

Pearsons's correlation	Cantril's ladder: lower scores = higher satisfaction	MMSE: lower score = more impairment	Barthel: lower score = more dependency	GDS-15: higher score = more 'depressed' responses	Uniscale: higher score = higher QOL judged by researchers
Life satisfaction total score	-0.403***	0.239**	0.214**	-0.554***	0.365***
Cantril's ladder		-0.028	-0.166*	0.409***	-0.347***
MMSE score		-0.023	0.232**	-0.103	0.336***
Barthel ADL Index				-0.292***	0.512***
GDS-15					-0.525***

N =					
Life satisfaction total score	170	186	185	185	186
Cantril's ladder		183	182	182	183
MMSE score			212	210	213
Barthel ADL Index				209	213
GDS-15					210

Notes:
*** significant at p ≤ 0.001.
** significant at p ≤ 0.01.
* significant at p ≤ 0.05.

Figure 5.7
Satisfaction with life today

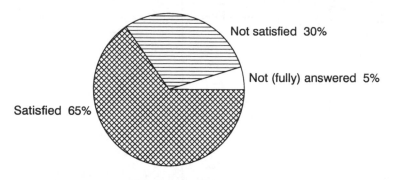

Not satisfied 30%

Not (fully) answered 5%

Satisfied 65%

Figure 5.8
Satisfaction with life as a whole

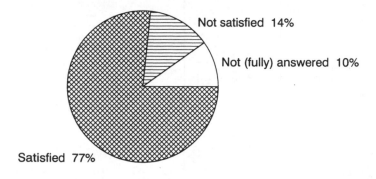

Not satisfied 14%

Not (fully) answered 10%

Satisfied 77%

with the residents' own view of the matter, measured by LSS total score or by Cantril's ladder. It should, however, be added that although a high level of significance was reached, the correlation coefficient ($r = 0.365$) was not very high.

When the binary satisfied / not satisfied variables are examined it is clear that a high proportion of the interviewed residents were satisfied with the various aspects of their lives (70.6 per cent satisfied overall, and on the separate domains ranging from 58.4 per cent (finance) to 74.8 per cent (social relationships)). Residents found it more difficult to answer questions on some domains. That 26.8 per cent of the residents found it impossible to answer the finance questions may reflect the fact that arrangements had been or were being made on their behalf. Many residents were quite content to let relatives deal with these matters and knew very little about their own finances. It is, perhaps, not surprising that health was the area in which residents were most likely to express dissatisfaction (a quarter of them did so) — in fact, given the extent of disability and dependency in this population it seems noteworthy that three-quarters of the interviewees were satisfied.

Figure 5.9 shows the association between dependency level and perceived quality of life in several life domains. A similar effect to that of depression can be observed, in that while high dependency reduces subjective ratings, individuals can still distinguish between life domains. For example, even the highly dependent residents are much happier about their social relationships than their finances or their health.

Figure 5.9
Life satisfaction and dependency level

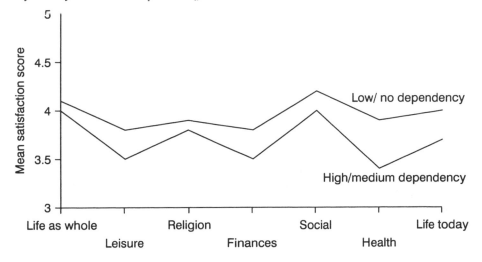

The living situation domain was the one which most clearly concerned the home and its services, including as it did, questions about privacy, independence, food quality, occupational opportunities and so on. Overall, 71.5 per cent of residents were satisfied with their living situation. There were however more dissatisfied responses to some individual questions than to others and these are summarised in Table 5.4. One-third of the residents were dissatisfied with the opportunities available for keeping themselves occupied in the home and relatively large numbers of people also reported dissatisfaction with opportunities for going out (26.9 per cent) and with their finances (25.6 per cent). Just over a quarter were dissatisfied with the amount of influence they had in the home. In fact it was clear from additional comments made in the interviews that very few residents thought they had any influence at all, seeing all decisions as being within the control of the staff. The three quarters who were satisfied may, therefore, have been saying not

Table 5.4
Individual questions on the 'living situation' domain of the LSS[a]

Item	% of respondents dissatisfied	Number of respondents dissatisfied[b]
How satisfied are you with:		
the living arrangements here?	13.7	27
the amount of independence you have here?	13.8	26
the amount of influence you have here?	25.9	41
living with the people you do?	18.7	34
the amount of privacy you have here?	12.2	24
the prospect of living here for a long time?	39.8	70
how well off you are financially?	25.6	44
the amount of money you have to spend on enjoyment?	23.3	38
the opportunities for getting out of the home?	26.9	42
the opportunities for keeping yourself occupied here in the home?	33.3	62
the quality and variety of food they serve?	13.7	24
being able to make your own drinks and snacks?	18.6	22
the time you have breakfast?	12.8	24
having your own things here with you in the home?	12.8	19

Notes:
a. As described in the text, the binary variables used here group 'very dissatisfied/mostly dissatisfied/mixed-uncertain' into one 'dissatisfied' response.
b. The number of missing responses varies, so the column on the right gives the actual number of dissatisfied respondents.

that they had influence but that they were content to have none or resigned to the fact. The highest proportion of dissatisfied responses was received in answer to the question about staying in the home for a long time. Just under 40 per cent were dissatisfied with the prospect of staying in the home for a long time. However, there were no associations found between dissatisfaction and home type, ownership sector or geographical location of the home.

Residents did express higher levels of perceived life satisfaction in some homes than in others. The mean LSS total score for each home was correlated with a number of variables which might be considered to have an impact on resident satisfaction. The N for these correlations was 30 (the homes) and Spearman's rho was used to test significance. This revealed no statistically significant correlations between mean total life satisfaction score in each home and any of the following:

- the seven Sheltered Care Environment Scale sub-scales ('mean for home' scores) (see further Chapter 7);
- the number of 'all carer' hours per occupied bed per day in the home;
- the number of care assistant hours per occupied bed per day;
- staff sickness rates;
- occupancy levels 1996 or 1997;
- the home's maximum weekly charge for care;
- the proportion of the home's resident population unable to walk, feed, use toilet, wash, incontinent, disoriented or with short-term memory loss.

The only environmental variable included in this exercise which showed a significant correlation with satisfaction was that relating to the proportion of residents in the home with persistent problem behaviours, such as wandering, screaming or being abusive (Spearman's rho $= -0.362$, $p = 0.05$). As usual when interpreting large numbers of correlations, caution is needed — this was the only significant result among the several relationships tested.

In summary

- Residents with depressive symptoms remained able to discriminate beween life domains in terms of their satisfaction with them.
- Overall well-being was higher for people with less cognitive impairment, less depression and less dependency.
- The reduction in the rating of overall well-being between the start and end of the interview was seen almost exclusively in depressed people.
- A researcher assessment of quality of life (the Spitzer Uniscale) was correlated moderately well with the residents' own view of their life quality.
- A high proportion of the interviewed residents were satisfied with the various aspects of their lives. Seventy-one per cent were satisfied overall; only 58 per cent were satisfied with finance but 75 per cent were satisfied with their social relationships. Even residents who were highly dependent were much more satisfied with their social relationships than their finances or their health.
- One-third of the residents were dissatisfied with the opportunities available for keeping themselves occupied in the home and over one-quarter also reported dissatisfaction with opportunities for going out (26.9 per cent), with their finances (25.6 per cent), and with the amount of influence they had in the home.
- The highest proportion of dissatisfied responses was received in answer to the question about staying in the home for a long time. Just under 40 per cent were dissatisfied with that prospect.

- Of a number of care environment variables examined, the only one which showed a significant correlation with dissatisfaction was that relating to the proportion of residents in the home with persistent problem behaviours.

6   The Experience of Care Staff

In a study like this one it was essential to find out as much as possible about the staff working in the homes. They are one of the most significant aspects of the care environment, their personalities and behaviour being very likely to affect residents' quality of life. Their intimate knowledge of the home also means that they are an invaluable source of information on the home generally, and on the communal life of residents.

Between six and nine months after the start of the project's fieldwork programme, questionnaires and Freepost envelopes for their confidential return were given to all the 1200 staff who worked in the 30 homes. Domestic, catering and maintenance staff were included as well as nursing or care staff. The questionnaire sought factual information about the respondent's background, training, experience, pay and conditions of service. It also included the GHQ-12, a job satisfaction scale, several scales designed to reflect the respondent's experience of being employed in the home, and the Sheltered Care Environment Scale.

The whole questionnaire was quite long and some response rate difficulty was anticipated. Two strategies were used in an attempt to alleviate this. Respondents who returned the questionnaire within one month were entered in a prize draw offering 40 prizes each worth £25 in supermarket tokens. In addition, by means of presentations to staff meetings, members of the research team took some trouble to inform staff about the project and try to give them a sense of involvement in it. Since it is known (Cartwright, 1978) that the one of the most significant factors in achieving good response to postal questionnaires is the perceived salience of the subject matter, it was hoped that this would overcome resistance to the length of the instrument.

Despite all this the overall response rate was a disappointing 37 per cent. This figure conceals enormous variation between homes, the individual home response rate ranging from 6 per cent to 84 per cent. Clearly the length of the questionnaire did not deter staff in all homes to a similar degree. The determining factor appeared to be the extent to which managers thought it important to involve staff in learning or thinking about their work. Response rates were very low in the few homes where it was impossible to arrange staff presentations at all, despite repeated requests over a period of three months and the willingness of team members to attend on more than one occasion, at evenings or weekends. In these homes, staff meetings of any kind appeared to be a rare occurrence. By contrast, the response was high in homes where management placed value on the presentation sessions and used them as training and general discussion opportunities. In the home with the 84 per cent response rate three separate sessions, including an evening one, were held at the request of the manager, who wanted all staff to have this training opportunity.

The low overall response is of greater significance for some parts of the questionnaire than for others. It does present a problem for analysis of the GHQ-12, since population estimates of the prevalence of mental distress may well be significantly affected (in either direction) by response rate bias. It is, however, unnecessary to have data from a large number of staff in order to establish the level of pay and conditions of service enjoyed by different grades of staff in the homes, or to gain a picture of the amount and content of in-service training provided. This chapter is concerned with data of this kind and there can be reasonable confidence in the limited effect of any response rate bias. Although they constitute a minority of the total staff, it must be remembered that the 440 respondents represent more than a third of the staff population of these 30 homes, and probably a larger number of care home staff than has been included in any similar survey in the UK.

The questionnaire respondents as a whole

The 440 respondents were drawn from the full range of occupational groups to be found in elderly care homes. The majority (53 per cent) were care or nursing assistants but there were significant numbers in other groups. The groups which included supervisory care staff — qualified nurses, sisters, care supervisors and deputy heads or 'second/third officers in charge' of residential homes — together constituted 24 per cent of the total.

Respondents were predominantly white (over 95 per cent), middle-aged (77 per cent aged 31 or over) and female (88 per cent). The vast majority (88 per cent) were permanent members of staff, rather than temporary or casual employees. Almost half (45 per cent) had been in their present jobs less than two years, but this was counterbalanced by some very long serving employees to produce a mean length of time in post of 50 months. Most of the staff in post less than two years had experience of similar work elsewhere. Overall, fewer than 15 per cent of respondents had less than two years' experience and the mean was 11 years, but there was a very wide range from nine months to 48 years. This was largely a part time workforce, working a mean of 27 hours each week. Sixty-one per cent worked for 30 hours a week or less.

A number of questionnaire items concerned pay and conditions of service. Since many people are reluctant to answer questions about money it was not surprising to find that some respondents refused to give this information. It was known in advance that supplying a choice of salary groups would be likely to produce a higher response. However, it was considered important to have exact information and few responses are necessary to produce comparative data on pay for similar staff in different homes or sectors. In the event 346 of the 440 did reveal their normal gross weekly pay and this information was used to compute the standard measure of an hourly rate of pay. Overall the mean gross rate of hourly pay was £5.16 and the most common (modal) rate of pay was £3.50 per hour. Forty-seven per cent were paid less than £4 and 65 per cent less than £5 per hour.[1]

Only 22 per cent of respondents belonged to an occupational pension scheme operated by their employer. Twelve per cent had no paid annual holiday and 34 per cent had less than 15 days a year. On the subject of sick leave entitlement there seemed to be some uncertainty. This question was unanswered or given a 'don't know' response in a large number of cases, leaving only 277 valid responses out of the possible 440. Those 277 were entitled to a mean of 40 days paid sick leave per annum (ranging from a minimum of no sick leave at all to a maximum of 182 days). Sick leave actually taken varied greatly between homes. This information was not obtained from the staff questionnaire but supplied from the home's records and thus more comprehensive in its coverage. Over a 12-month period immediately prior to the study the mean sick leave per member of staff in the study homes was 10.1 days (std.dev. 11.9).

Table 6.1 shows the qualifications held, and job-related courses of study undertaken by respondents. The majority (59 per cent) had no job-related qualifications of any kind. There were 81 (19 per cent of the total) with various nursing qualifications and 40 NVQ participants. Most of the latter had attained levels 1 and 2 with only three people having levels 3 or 4. It is of note that a recent study of training needs of care staff carried out in care homes in North West England found a higher percentage of care and nursing assistant staff qualified to NVQ level 2 (Bagley et al., 2001). Between 17 per cent and 20 per cent of care and nursing assistant staff were qualified to NVQ level 2,

---

1 It should be recalled that the questionnaires were completed in summer 1997.

Table 6.1
Staff main qualifications and job-related courses

	Number of respondents	Percentage of respondents
No job-related qualification	256	59.0
RGN	38	8.8
RMN	15	3.5
EN(Gen)	19	4.4
EN(Mental)	1	0.2
Nursing degree/diploma	8	1.8
CQSW /DIPSW	2	0.5
CSS	3	0.7
ENB elderly care courses (various)	6	1.4
Chiropody/physiotherapy	2	0.5
Care NVQ levels 1/2	37	8.5
Care NVQ levels 3/4	3	0.7
Other care courses	16	3.7
Catering courses	17	3.9
Secretarial/admin.	5	1.2
Business/management	3	0.7
Other qualifications/courses	3	0.7
Total	434	100

compared to just 8.5 per cent of staff in this study. A further 22 to 26 per cent of the care staff were actively working towards this level of training. However, there were similarities between the studies with respect to the proportion of staff qualified to NVQ level 3 and above. Training to level 3 was rare, with less than one per cent of staff qualified to this level, in both this and the Training Needs Study.

National minimum standards for care homes introduced in April 2002 specify that 50 per cent of staff employed in continuing care homes will have an NVQ level 2 qualification by 2005, as required by the Care Standards Act (2000). It is therefore encouraging that a study undertaken in 2001 has shown a larger proportion of care staff reaching NVQ level 2, indicating that there has been modest progress. However, this rate of increase needs to be maintained or improved in order to achieve this target.

Ownership sectors compared — all respondents

Three home ownership sectors are represented in the data and it is possible to compare the responses of staff in privately owned, local authority and voluntary homes. The last group included former local authority homes now owned by an independent non-profit organisation.

There was a statistically significant association between age group and ownership sector ($\chi^2(4) = 12.667$, $p = 0.013$), with fewer respondents in local authority homes who were aged under 30. There were no significant differences in sex or ethnic origin, or in the proportions of permanent as opposed to temporary or casual staff. The median length of time in the current job, at five years, was much longer for the local authority staff than the other two groups. For local authority staff median length of relevant work experience was ten years, compared with nine years for private and seven years for voluntary homes staff.

Table 6.2 shows summary statistics for normal weekly hours worked, hourly pay rate and annual sick leave allowance, all broken down by ownership sector. In the private sector there was a much wider range of hourly pay rates. The median pay rate was lowest in the private sector, slightly higher in the voluntary sector and quite a lot higher for local authority respondents.

This table illustrates a large difference in the annual sick leave allowance given to staff. As high as at the third quartile level, private sector respondents had no paid sick leave at all; voluntary sector and local authority respondents

Table 6.2

All staff questionnaire respondents: pay, hours, sick leave, by ownership sector (1997 figures)

					Interquartile range	
	Valid N	Median	Min.	Max.	25%	75%
Private						
Hours worked per week	166	30.00	1.00	47.00	18.0	37.00
Gross pay per hour	131	3.64	0.00	27.78	03.1	6.03
Annual sick leave						
allowance on full pay	131	0.00	0.00	180.0	0.00	0.00
Voluntary						
Hours worked per week	196	25.00	7.00	42.00	20.00	31.75
Gross pay per hour	163	3.80	1.24	10.86	3.45	4.80
Annual sick leave						
allowance on full pay	111	0.00	0.00	180.0	0.00	90.00
Local authority						
Hours worked per week	61	28.00	10.00	39.00	22.00	39.00
Gross pay per hour	50	5.17	0.00	10.20	4.39	6.00
Annual sick leave allowance						
on full pay	43	180.00	0.00	182.0	90.00	180.00

had 90 days and 180 days respectively. Of the respondents who knew whether or not they had any sick leave entitlement, in private homes 84.7 per cent had none at all, compared with 50.5 per cent in voluntary and 11.6 per cent in local authority homes. This may have had some connection with the different level of staff sickness reported by managers for the year prior to the study. The median number of sick days per staff member in the private sector was 2.77 and in voluntary and local authority homes 10.23, a difference which was statistically significant (Mann Whitney, p = 0.001).

Respondents employed by local authorities were also more favourably treated in the matter of occupational pension provision, 70.5 per cent being members of an occupational scheme, compared with 21 per cent of voluntary and only 6 per cent of private home respondents. There was a significant association between membership of an occupational pension scheme and ownership sector ($\chi^2(2) = 108.3$, p < 0.001).

Care and nursing assistants as a separate group

In matters of pay, conditions of service and in-service training it seems sensible to consider separately the 230 respondents who were employed as care or

Table 6.3
Care assistants only: pay, hours, sick leave, by ownership sector (1997 figures)

					Interquartile range	
	Valid N	Median	Min.	Max.	25%	75%
Private						
Hours worked per week	67	34.00	4.00	46.00	21.00	37.00
Gross pay per hour	54	3.15	1.24	23.10	2.85	3.46
Annual sick leave						
allowance on full pay	49	0.00	0.00	14.00	0.00	0.00
Voluntary						
Hours worked per week	116	25.00	9.00	42.00	20.00	31.75
Gross pay per hour	96	3.62	1.24	9.60	3.39	4.48
Annual sick leave						
allowance on full pay	61	0.00	0.00	180.0	0.00	28.00
Local authority						
Hours worked per week	42	23.50	10.00	39.00	22.00	35.00
Gross pay per hour	35	5.51	0.00	10.20	4.79	6.00
Annual sick leave allowance						
on full pay	32	180.00	0.00	182.0	54.00	180.00

nursing assistants, since the content of the job and the attributes required of staff who do it are broadly similar in all care homes.

For this group of staff the median gross hourly rate of pay was £3.57. The range was from no pay at all to £23.00 per hour, but both figures represent very unusual extremes — a volunteer and a relative of the owner.

Table 6.3 displays summary statistics similar to those shown in Table 6.2. The pattern observed for all respondents is repeated here except that slightly fewer weekly hours were worked by local authority care assistants. The median and third quartile figures for all three variables provide an interesting basis for comparison, the contrast between the third quartile values for pay and sick leave between private and local authority homes being particularly pronounced. The wide difference between sectors in occupational pension coverage was similar to that seen for respondents as a whole.

Staff were asked for details of any in-service training they had received in their present job and a summary of the answers given by nursing and care assistants is shown in Table 6.4. It is clear that even basic in-service training was by no means a universal practice. Just under half the assistants had been

Table 6.4

Nursing/care assistants only: in-service training received in current job

Subject area	Percentage who have done training in this area during present employment
Basic care skills, (including lifting and handling, basic hygiene)	49.1
Safety (health and safety procedures, fire safety, toxic substances, first aid)	39.6
Catering/food hygiene	13.9
Borderline nursing/ care procedures (e.g. pressure area care, catheter care, medication, drugs, aids, nutrition)	10.9
The physical problems of residents	9.1
'Our way of doing things' (customer care, complaints procedures, dealing with residents and relatives, induction training)	8.7
The psychiatric/psychological problems of residents (including dementia care, depression, dealing with problem behaviour, emotional care of the dying)	7.8
Care planning	5.2
Technical nursing procedures (e.g. gastroscopy, wound care, pain control, resuscitation)	3.5
Personal/interpersonal skill development	2.6
Management development/supervision skills	2.2
Administration/computer use/book-keeping/accounts	1.3

trained in basic care skills, including lifting and handling; and fewer than 40 per cent had done safety training of any kind. While many of these staff had prior experience in other homes, this kind of in-service training is often site-specific or needs regular refresher sessions.

It was also noteworthy that very few of the assistants said they had received training to help them understand the physical or psychological problems of residents, however broadly defined. So few respondents reported training in psychiatric or psychological problems generally, in dementia and its behavioural implications, in recognising or managing depression, or in emotional care of the dying that any training of the kind was grouped as one broad category. Only 7.8 per cent of the assistants reported receiving any in-service training of this kind.

The data were examined to see whether there were any ownership sector differences in the training of care and nursing assistants. There were no differences, with the sole exception of training in care planning ($\chi^2(2) = 12.02$, $p = 0.002$). The only in-service training on care planning reported by care or nursing assistants took place in the voluntary sector.

The experience of daily working life — job satisfaction and mental health

The Staff Questionnaire contained a number of scales measuring the job satisfaction of respondents and their experience of particular aspects of their work environment, as well as a measure of mental distress (particularly psychiatric 'caseness'). The instruments used are described in Chapter 3 but to aid interpretation, Table 6.5 contains a summary of the scales adopted from the work of Borrill et al. (1996) in their study of mental health in the staff of NHS Trusts ('the NHS workforce survey'). Eight of these scales were used in that study to measure 'work related factors' which might be associated with mental health. These were: job autonomy and control; role clarity; work demands; feedback; leader support; influence over decisions; social support; and role conflict. Three further scales measured aspects of the organisational climate as experienced by respondents, and one measured the respondent's commitment to the job. These were: formality; effort; initiative; and job commitment. Each scale contained between four and six items scored on a five-point 'Likert' scale. Psychological distress was measured using the General Health Questionnaire in its short version (GHQ-12, Goldberg and Williams, 1988), and the Job Satisfaction Scale was that devised by Warr et al. (1979).

It must be recalled that the overall response rate to this questionnaire was 37 per cent and that there was considerable between-home variation in response. Non-response bias must always be a concern in using measures like the General Health Questionnaire since there may well be reasons for non-

Table 6.5
Work related factors

Scale name	Direction of measurement
1. Job autonomy and control	high score = much individual choice about how work
2. Role clarity (called ambiguity in the NHS Workforce Survey)	high score = little ambiguity/much clarity about job requirements
3. Work demands	high score = high perceived level of work demands/pressure
4. Feedback	high score = much feedback about individual's job performance
5. Leader support	high score = high level of support/ encouragement from superior
6. Influence over decisions	high score = individual has much influence over work decisions
7. Social support	high score = individual receives much supoprt from co-workers
8. Role conflict	high score = individual experiences much role conflict
Organisational climate	
1. Formality	high score = a climate of informality
2. Effort	high score = staff generally put extra effort into their work
3. Initiative (called 'autonomy' in the NHS Workforce Survey)	high score = a climate in which staff are allowed to use initiative
4. Job commitment	high score = high level of commitment

response that have to do with the existence of psychological distress. As Goldberg and Williams (1988) report, it is unclear whether non-respondents are more or less likely to be high GHQ scorers. In this study there did appear to be some relationship between the within-home response rate and the enthusiasm with which managers involved their staff in discussion about the project, but the relationship is not a clear one and there are no reasons to conclude that staff in homes with managers less enthusiastic about research will suffer from more symptoms of mental distress.

Despite the doubts about non-response bias, the 440 respondents did constitute 37 per cent of the whole staff population of the 30 homes, and in several homes included the majority of the home's staff. It is, therefore, reasonable to report the GHQ data for the group of respondents, and to look at the ways in which their scores are related to other factors while taking care to avoid drawing unwarranted inferences about the wider population of residential and nursing home staff generally.

The GHQ was scored in two ways, described by Goldberg and Williams (1988) as the 'GHQ method' (0–0–1–1) and the 'Likert method' (0–1–2–3). Using the GHQ scoring method with a threshold of 3/4 it is possible to divide respondents into 'cases' and 'non-cases', the former being those who exhibit symptoms of psychological distress to an extent such that a psychiatrist would probably consider intervention appropriate. Various threshold scores have been reported in independent studies (Goldberg and Williams, 1988). The threshold of 3/4 is a conservative one (i.e. unlikely to classify non-cases as cases) and has been chosen in part so as to facilitate comparison with the 'caseness' estimates obtained in the NHS workforce survey.

Overall, 15.7 per cent of respondents were classified as cases. This was much lower than the rate reported for NHS staff of 26.8 per cent (Wall et al., 1997), and more closely in line with general population survey findings such as the British Household Panel Survey (Taylor et al., 1995) used for comparison by Wall et al. (1997), which reports an overall case rate of 17.8 per cent.

The present study findings are of interest when compared to those of the NHS workforce survey because they concern occupational groups which are in many respects similar. The surveyed NHS staff included many more groups of staff but two occupational groups are broadly comparable between the two studies. 'Nurses' in the NHS workforce survey included nursing staff of all grades and the reported caseness of 28.5 per cent can, therefore, be compared with 17.2 per cent among all nursing and care staff in the 30 homes. The percentage of cases (20.1 per cent) in NHS ancillary staff compares with 14.9 per cent for domestic, maintenance and catering staff in the homes. There are many reasons for treating this comparison with extreme caution. The response rate problem has been mentioned, but there must be added to that the very different sample size and sampling method of the two studies. The NHS workforce survey occupational group figures also incorporate controls for factors such as age and marital status. However the difference in case rates is such as to suggest that the care home workers were more like the general population and less like the NHS workers in this respect.

As a simple check on the differences in prevalence (if any) between staff in homes with different within-home response rates, separate case percentages were calculated for three sub-groups of respondents who were in homes in three different response bands. In homes with a lower than 25 per cent response rate, 14.1 per cent of respondents were cases, in homes with between 25 and 50 per cent response, 15.8 per cent were cases, and in homes with better than a 50 per cent response rate, 16.3 per cent were cases. There was no statistically significant association between caseness and being in a home within a particular response rate band (χ^2 (2) = 1.81, p = 0.9).

Personal characteristics, work related factors and psychological distress

In this sample of care home staff, GHQ caseness was significantly associated with:

- Having experienced any major life event (for example marriage, serious illness, divorce) during the preceding six months ($\chi^2(1) = 5.38$, p = 0.027). Of those who had experienced major life events 23.7 per cent were above the case threshold, compared with 13.8 per cent of those who had not.
- Being in a lower age group. Of staff aged under 30, 28.9 per cent were 'cases' compared with 14.2 per cent of staff aged 31 to 50 and 9 per cent of staff over 51. There were statistically significant differences between staff aged under 30 and those in both the other age groups, those aged 31–50 (Mann-Whitney U = 8734.5, p =0.002), and those aged over 51 (Mann-Whitney U = 4742.5, p < 0.001).

Caseness was not significantly associated with:

- Job category — either across the range of jobs or when staff were divided into two groups depending on whether or not they had supervisory responsibility for others.
- Employment sector, whether private/voluntary/local authority or nursing/ residential.

Thus, psychological distress was more likely in younger people and those having experienced a recent life event.

Correlations between the eight work-related factor scales and mental distress as measured by the GHQ-12 were examined, using a Pearson's one-tailed test. Seven of the eight factors (all except feedback') were significantly correlated with GHQ score, at the .01 level, all in the expected direction, higher GHQ score (more mental distress) being significantly correlated with:

- more work demands;
- more role conflict;
- less role clarity;
- less leader support;
- less social support from work colleagues;
- less influence over work decisions; and
- less job autonomy and control.

It should be added that although the correlations were statistically significant the coefficients were not very high — the highest being 'work demands' at 0.376; and that causation cannot be inferred from this. It is impossible to say, for example, whether higher demands at work result in psychological distress or being psychologically distressed makes work appear to be more demanding.

Higher GHQ scores were also significantly correlated (at the .01 level — Pearson's two tailed test) with:

- a climate in which workers put less effort into their work;
- a climate in which workers are encouraged to use their initiative; and
- a high level of job commitment.

Again, although the correlations were statistically significant, the correlations were relatively low, ranging from 0.275 to 0.165. Also, it was interesting to note that both undemanding environments and places where staff had high levels of commitment and demonstrated their initiative, were similarly likely to have staff who experienced high levels of distress.

Some associations with job satisfaction

The relationships between job satisfaction and a number of factors were explored using Kruskall-Wallis tests, followed by Mann-Whitney U tests on each individual pairing. A difference between the three ownership sectors turned out to be a difference between the private and voluntary sectors (Mann-Whitney $U = 11481$, $p = 0.001$). At 4.9 and 4.87 respectively the median job satisfaction scores in voluntary and local authority homes were significantly higher than the private homes' 4.6, where job satisfaction appeared to be lowest.

Job satisfaction for the under-30 age group was significantly lower than for either of the older groups. (Under 30 and 31–50 age group, Mann-Whitney $U = 6354$, $p < 0.001$; under 30 and over 51 age group, Mann-Whitney $U = 2912$, $p < 0.001$). It will be recalled that the proportion of GHQ-identified 'cases' was higher in this younger group, which appears consistent with the finding of lower job satisfaction.

In summary

- Staff questionnaires were returned by 37 per cent of home staff, although there was considerable variation between the homes, ranging from 6 per cent to 84 per cent response rate. All types of employees were involved, including domestic, catering, maintenance staff and voluntary workers.

- Mean length of time in current post was 50 months, although for staff in local authority homes this was much longer than for private or voluntary home staff.
- Median pay rate and annual sick leave allowance was lowest in the private sector. While the majority of local authority home staff were in occupational pension schemes, few staff in the private or voluntary sectors had similar cover.
- Nursing staff and care assistants had received little in-service training in their present jobs. Less than half had received basic care skills training including lifting and handling, and less than two-fifths had done safety training. Less than 10 per cent had received training in any aspects of psychiatric or psychological problems including dementia, in the recognition or management of depression, or in terminal care.
- Using the GHQ-12 as a measure of psychological distress, 15.7 per cent of staff respondents were classified as 'cases', lower than that reported for NHS staff (26.8 per cent). GHQ 'caseness' was significantly associated with having experienced a major life event or being in a lower age group, and was related to a number of work-related factors, in particular 'higher demands at work'.
- Job satisfaction was significantly higher in voluntary and local authority homes, and among older staff members.

7 The Culture of the Care Environment: the Sheltered Care Environment Scale

In this chapter, an attempt is made to identify the different care environments of the homes in the study. The Sheltered Care Environment Scale (Moos and Lemke, 1984, 1992) was included in the Staff Questionnaire. As described in Chapter 3, this scale is designed to measure the social environment of the home and contains sub-scales measuring seven dimensions: *cohesion, conflict, independence, self-disclosure, organization, resident influence* and *physical comfort*. The sub-scales, their content and direction of measurement are summarised in Table 7.1.

Table 7.2 displays the mean sub-scale scores for each of the 30 homes with the exception of one home where only one staff member completed the scale. Scores have been computed for one home where only four staff responded and these data should be treated with caution. For all the other homes the response threshold recommended by Moos and Lemke (1984) was met — five or more respondents per home.

Table 7.3 sets the Sheltered Care Environment Scale sub-scale data in the context of some other studies in residential and nursing homes, in the UK and in the US. The scores for the study homes were closer to those for Netten's (1993) UK residential homes than to the American facilities on some sub-scales, but not on all of them. Netten's finding of significantly higher conflict (extent to which residents express anger and criticism) in her UK homes was not repeated here but the apparent UK/US difference in the independence scores (extent to which resident independence is encouraged) is maintained. It might have been thought that the independence scores would be lower in the nursing homes, with their more dependent resident populations.

Similar research carried out in the US investigating quality of life of residents in assisted living homes used four sub-scales of the SCES: *cohesion;*

Table 7.1
The structure of the Sheltered Care Environment Scale

SCES Sub-scale	Dimension measured	Direction of score
Cohesion	Staff report extent of helpfulness of staff to residents and between residents	high = more helpfulness
Conflict	Staff report extent to which residents express anger, criticise each other and home	high = more anger/ criticism
Self disclosure	Staff report extent to which residents openly express feelings and concerns	high = more open expression
Independence	Staff report extent to which independence is encouraged in residents	high = more encouragement of independence
Resident influence	Staff report extent of residents' influence on rules and policies of the home; their freedom from restrictive regulations	high = more resident influence
Organization	Staff report importance of order in the home; clarity and predictability of rules and routine	high = more organised
Physical comfort	Staff report extent to which physical environment offers comfort, privacy. Pleasant surroundings	high = more comfort or pleasantness

conflict; independence; and *resident influence* (Mitchell and Kemp, 2000). However in this case, the sub-scale scores were gained from interviews with residents themselves. The average scores for the four social climate measures differed in many ways from those of the present study. Although their mean score for cohesion (mean 58.3) was very similar to those for 'all homes' and 'residential homes only' in this present study (shown in Table 7.3), scores for *conflict* were very much lower than in the present study (mean 34.9) indicating less conflict. Conversely, scores for *independence* (mean 26.4) and *resident influence* (mean 41.2) were also much lower than in this study, indicating an environment that is less encouraging of resident independence and one of less resident influence.

One cannot infer from this whether these differences reflect variation in the care environment of long-stay homes between the two countries, or whether they can be accounted for by the fact that residents themselves completed the scale, revealing different opinions from those of care staff. Of the latter suggestion, it would appear that the scores of the US study (Mitchell and Kemp, 2000) also vary somewhat from the US residential homes study (Moos and Lemke, 1992), shown in Table 7.3. This may indicate that disparities in

Table 7.2
Mean 'within home' SCES subscale scores*

Home	Cohesion	Conflict	Indepen-dence	Self-disclosure	Organiz-ation	Resident Influence	Physical Comfort
a	51.39	56.94	31.94	56.94	48.61	59.72	88.89
b	66.67	75.55	44.44	60.00	62.22	53.33	88.89
c	64.29	66.67	37.30	52.38	53.17	63.49	77.78
d	59.65	49.71	35.09	46.78	49.12	70.18	79.53
e	58.02	59.88	33.95	73.46	58.64	66.05	74.07
f	77.78	55.56	80.00	48.89	60.00	82.00	80.00
g	79.71	62.31	42.51	68.60	62.32	77.78	78.74
h	52.14	58.12	33.33	68.38	58.12	60.68	75.50
i	54.76	66.67	26.98	58.73	43.65	69.84	77.78
j	61.11	68.98	34.26	56.02	53.24	68.52	68.52
k	73.74	61.62	33.33	74.75	61.62	73.74	79.80
l	53.09	58.02	32.10	59.26	54.32	64.20	71.60
m	66.67	72.22	30.56	73.61	59.72	84.72	79.17
n	48.48	62.63	37.37	62.62	50.51	78.79	67.68
o	42.31	72.65	34.62	59.40	51.71	50.43	76.07
p	52.78	62.22	26.67	48.06	59.17	66.11	64.44
q	64.02	51.85	31.22	59.26	52.38	67.72	79.37
r	41.11	78.89	32.22	66.11	56.11	72.22	61.11
s	72.22	50.00	48.15	68.52	61.11	64.81	77.78
t	71.72	44.44	46.46	72.73	67.68	83.84	91.92
u	71.43	60.32	42.86	73.02	58.73	74.60	74.60
v (n=4)	33.33	69.44	16.67	55.56	36.11	58.33	61.11
w	42.86	61.90	31.75	39.68	49.21	61.90	71.43
x	59.26	77.78	33.33	61.11	53.70	77.78	75.96
y	44.44	68.25	15.87	52.38	55.56	53.97	68.25
z	66.67	73.02	22.22	64.29	52.38	71.43	69.05
aa			Not computed: (n=1)				
bb	61.50	51.94	35.66	54.52	61.50	53.23	78.81
cc	70.94	57.27	59.83	59.83	60.68	75.21	78.63
dd	62.96	62.96	29.63	57.41	57.41	75.93	74.07

Note: * n (number of staff respondents) ≥ 5 unless otherwise stated.

scores may occur depending upon who completes the scale. This again illustrates that measures of care environments may produce different outcomes depending upon whose views are sought.

There were statistically significant differences between this study's nursing and residential home groups only in the scores for *self-disclosure* (extent to which residents express feelings openly) and *resident influence* (extent of resident influence on home policies and rules) (Mann-Whitney, p <0.001). Figures 7.1 and 7.2 illustrate the otherwise broadly similar score profiles of the two groups of homes.

Table 7.3
Sheltered Care Environment Scale — comparison with other studies

| SCES sub-scales | Quality of life Study | | | | | | UK residential homes[a] (13 homes) | | US residential homes[b] (55 homes) | | US nursing homes[c] (127 homes) | | US assisted living[d] (55 facilities) | |
| | All homes (30 homes) | | Nursing homes only (12 homes) | | Residential homes only (17 homes) | | | | | | | | | |
	Mean	SD	Mean	SD	Mean	SD	Mean	SD	Mean	SD	Mean	SD	Mean	SD
Cohesion	59	26	56	26	62	26	52	28	75	14	69	11	58	23
Conflict	62	23	59	24	65	23	76	17	49	20	64	12	35	29
Independence	34	20	32	20	37	20	26	20	55	15	53	9	26	20
Self-disclosure	60	24	56	24	64	22	65	22	60	15	63	10	–	–
Organisation	56	16	56	16	57	16	53	26	73	14	60	12	–	–
Resident influence	67	20	62	19	72	20	71	21	60	16	60	9	41	22
Physical comfort	75	18	75	18	74	17	67	13	80	12	67	12	–	–

Notes:
a. Netten (1993).
b. Moos and Lemke (1992).
c. Moos and Lemke (1992).
d. Mitchell and Kemp (2000).

Figure 7.1

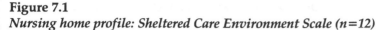

Nursing home profile: Sheltered Care Environment Scale (n=12)

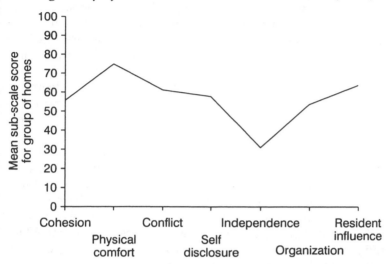

Figure 7.2

Residential home profile: Sheltered Care Environment Scale (n=17)

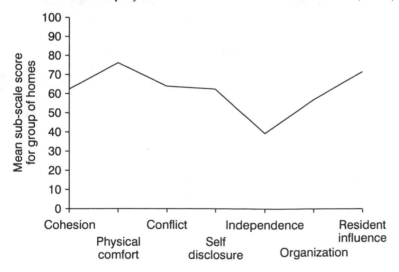

The originators of the Sheltered Care Environment Scale devised a social climate typology which uses the seven sub-scales to classify homes by regime type. Derived from cluster analysis of data from 235 residential institutions in the US, the Timko and Moos (1991b) classification describes six home types as *supportive, self-directed; supportive, well organised; open conflict; suppressed conflict; emergent-positive* and *unresponsive.*

Using a simpler typology, namely Booth's (1985) three-way classification of homes, Netten (1993) carried out a cluster analysis of 13 residential homes using Sheltered Care Environment Scale data. Booth's homes are classified according to their 'regime types'. Homes described as *positive* are those which allow residents to act or choose things for themselves, and show a 'positive approach to residents' capabilities', thus permitting them a high degree of freedom and choice. Homes described as *mixed* are those which are regarded as having 'multiple regimes', where presence of freedom and choice in some areas are counterbalanced almost equally by regulation and control in other areas. Homes described as *restrictive* have low freedom and choice, and show a narrow or restricted attitude to residents' capabilities, limiting their freedom to act or think for themselves. In Netten's sample, positive homes were those with high scores for the sub-scales on *resident influence, independence, cohesion* and *conflict*. Subject to confirmation by other research it was suggested that it might be possible to classify as *positive* homes with scores greater than 30 for *independence* and greater than 80 for *resident influence*. Homes scoring less than 12 for *independence* might be classified as *restrictive*.

Application of these threshold scores to the homes in this study was not productive. Only three homes had *independence* and *resident influence* scores higher than 30 and 80 respectively so that, in Netten's suggested terms, they would be classified as *positive*. None of the homes in this study had independence scores lower than the 12 required to classify a home as *restrictive*. The homes in this study were, however, sufficiently varied to make it unhelpful simply to describe all but three of them as *mixed*.

Similarly to the treatment of the data used by Netten, Cluster Analysis was used to look for patterns which would justify grouping the homes. As a first step the individual sub-scale scores for the 414 Sheltered Care Environment Scale respondents were subjected to Principal Components analysis using Varimax rotation. Initial statistics revealed that *cohesion* (helpfulness of staff to resident and between residents) accounted for 39.8 per cent of the variance and *conflict* for a further 20.2 per cent. Two factors were extracted. Grouped with *cohesion* were *self-disclosure, independence* and *resident influence*. The second factor contained high positive loadings for *physical comfort* and *organization* with a negative loading for *conflict*.

Cluster analysis was then carried out (K-Means Clustering with classification and iteration) using the 'mean for home' scores on just the two scale variables, *cohesion* and *conflict*. Groups of from two to five were examined for distinctiveness in terms of the *cohesion/conflict* scores; compared with researchers' experience of the homes over two years of regular fieldwork visits; and tested for the extent to which there were significant between-group differences in the other Sheltered Care Environment Scale sub-scale scores. At this stage three clusters appeared which seemed to define groups of homes to the reasonable satisfaction of the researcher doing the clustering exercise and corresponded in general terms to the *restrictive / mixed / positive* typology of Booth (1985).

- Cluster 1 homes had low *cohesion* and high *conflict* scores. Whether or not the appropriate descriptive term for this group is *restrictive* it is the case that the researcher had doubts about the quality of most of the homes in this group. With one exception, these were homes they would not personally have chosen for a relative's care.
- Cluster 2 homes had middle-range scores for both these key sub-scales and can fairly be described as *mixed*. The researcher would have put one of

Table 7.4
The three home clusters and the other five SCES sub-scales

Three clusters cohesion/conflict only			N	Mean rank[*]	p
Self disclosure					
	restrictive	1	10	11.80	
	mixed	2	9	16.39	ns
	positive	3	10	16.95	
	Total		29		
Independence					
	restrictive	1	10	10.30	
	mixed	2	9	12.67	0.006
	positive	3	10	21.80	
	Total		29		
Resident influence					
	restrictive	1	10	9.90	
	mixed	2	9	16.61	ns
	positive	3	10	18.65	
	Total		29		
Organisation					
	restrictive	1	10	10.10	
	mixed	2	9	13.94	0.017
	positive	3	10	20.85	
	Total		29		
Physical comfort					
	restrictive	1	10	8.75	
	mixed	2	9	14.61	0.003
	positive	3	10	21.60	
	Total		29		

Note: * Kruskall Wallis test.

these nine homes in the 'top' group and one in the 'bottom', but in general would have described them as being of average or indifferent quality.

• Cluster 3 homes had high *cohesion* and low *conflict* scores and the researcher thought that perhaps they warranted the description of *positive*. Of these ten homes there were two she would not have rated so highly.

Gibbs and Sinclair (1992a) have shown that 'expert' judges often disagree about home quality, and this occasion was no exception. There were different views among the research team as to the appropriateness of the categorisation of some homes. There was agreement about a number of the homes in Clusters 1 and 3, but a number of Cluster 2 homes and some in 1 and 3 would have been reallocated by one or more researchers. This serves only to illustrate the extent to which Cluster Analysis ultimately depends on the interpretation put on the groups, and the fact that one person's ideal care home will not appear that way to everybody. With that considerable caution it is, nevertheless, an interesting exercise to see how the clusters based upon the degree of *cohesion* and *conflict* sorted the homes.

Table 7.4 displays the rankings for a series of Kruskall-Wallis tests designed to examine the extent to which there are significant differences between these three groups of homes on the other five sub-scale scores. There are statistically significant differences between the groups in *independence* ($p = 0.006$), *organization* ($p = 0.017$) and *physical comfort* ($p = 0.003$), but not in *self-disclosure* ($p = 0.337$) or *resident influence* ($p = 0.056$). Figures 7.3 to 7.5 show group profiles for the three clusters of homes, on all the Sheltered Care Environment Scale sub-scales.

Figure 7.3
Cluster 1 profile: Sheltered Care Environment Scale (n=10)

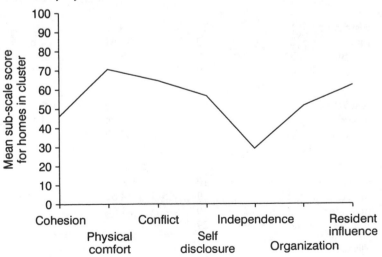

Figure 7.4
Cluster 2 profile: Sheltered Care Environment Scale (n=9)

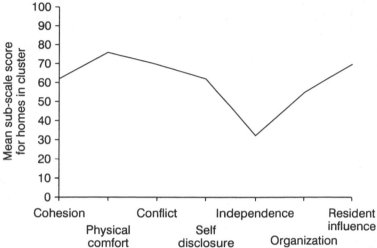

Figure 7.5
Cluster 3 profile: Sheltered Care Environment Scale (n=10)

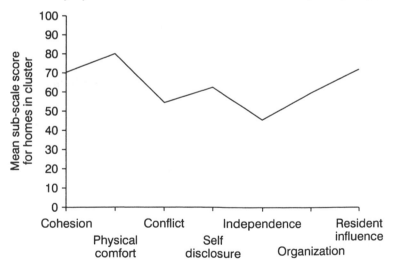

The data were explored for possible relationships between the homes' cluster membership and a number of other variables. Kruskall-Wallis tests were used to investigate relationships between the clustering and a number of staff or home-related factors, and the 'work related factors', organisational climate, job satisfaction and staff mental distress measures described in Chapter 6. There were no statistically significant differences between the three clusters and staff or home-related factors, nor were any statistically significant differences were found between the clusters and the work-related factors. The variables included in these analyses are shown in Table 7.5. Thus the division into the three clusters cuts across the distinction between nursing and residential homes and does not appear to be related either to the dependency level of the resident populations or to staffing density.

Statistically significant 'between-cluster' differences were, however, found in five of the work and organisational variables (illustrated in Table 6.5) namely:

- work demands (p = 0.001);
- role conflict (p = 0.016).

Table 7.5
Variables showing a non-significant relationship between the three clusters (Kruskall-Wallis test)

Staff and home related factors	Work related factors
• size of home (total beds)	• job autonomy and control
• number of 'all carer' hours per week per occupied bed	• role clarity
• number of care assistant hours per week per occupied bed	• feedback
• number of domestic / catering staff hours per week per occupied bed	• leader support
• maximum charge per week	• influence over decisions
• percentage occupancy July 1996	• social support
• percentage occupancy July 1997	• formality of climate
• percentage of residents unable to feed self without help	• initiative promoting climate
• percentage of residents unable to use WC without help	• staff mental distress (GHQ, Likert scored)
• percentage of residents unable to walk indoors without help	
• percentage of residents unable to wash hands and face without help	
• percentage of residents persistently incontinent	
• percentage of residents persistently disoriented	
• percentage of residents with persistent short-term memory problems	
• percentage of residents with persistent problem behaviours	

Figure 7.6
The three home clusters and 'work demands' (n=429)

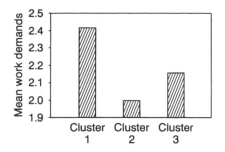

Figure 7.9
The three home clusters and 'job commitment' (n=427)

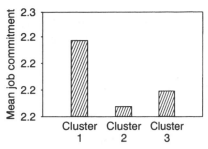

Figure 7.7
The three home clusters and 'role conflict' (n=429)

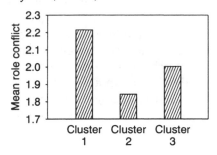

Figure 7.10
The three home clusters and 'job satisfaction' (n=400)

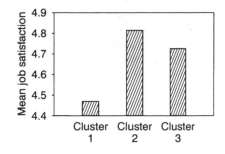

Figure 7.8
The three home clusters and 'high effort climate' (n=427)

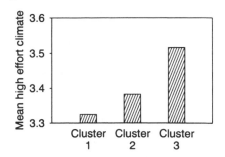

- effort climate (p = 0.006);
- job commitment (p = 0.006); and
- job satisfaction (p = 0.001).

These are illustrated in Figures 7.6 to 7.10. Compared with both the other groups, Cluster 1 homes (the ones seen as being of lower quality) had scores reflecting significantly higher work demands and role conflict, with significantly lower job satisfaction and a climate of lower effort, or demands upon staff. Cluster 3 homes (the higher quality ones) had scores which fell between the other two groups for work demands, role conflict and job satisfaction — though in the latter case the score was much higher than Cluster 1. This higher quality group of homes reported the highest 'effort climate', or staff demands. Cluster 2 presented a mixed picture, combining job satisfaction higher than in Cluster 3 with low work demands, low role conflict and a climate of relatively low effort. At first sight the scores for 'job commitment' seem surprising. In Cluster 1, with its high work demands, high role conflict and low job satisfaction, commitment is high. That workers should be committed to remaining in the job appears inconsistent until the content of the commitment questions is examined. This scale includes questions asking whether respondents would leave the home if it was not doing well, or if they were offered a little more money elsewhere. It may be that the staff working in Cluster 1 homes were prepared to put up with working in a demanding job which offered little satisfaction because it offered convenience in terms of location or hours — or because they saw themselves as having few other options.

In summary

- As part of the staff questionnaire, home staff completed the Sheltered Care Environment Scale, which measures the social environment of the home. The scores for the study homes were more similar to those for Netten's (1993) UK residential homes study than those conducted in American nursing or residential homes.
- Cluster analysis revealed three clusters which appeared to correspond in general terms to the *restrictive/ mixed/ positive* typology of Booth (1985). Cluster 1 (*restrictive*) homes had low *cohesion* and high *conflict* scores; Cluster 2 (*mixed*) had mid-range scores for both sub-scales, and Cluster 3 (*positive*) homes had high *cohesion* and low *conflict* scores. Although there was general agreement for a number of homes, they were not all clustered in accordance with researchers' (personal) ratings of the homes.
- There were no statistically significant differences between the three clusters on a number of home and work-related factors, such as size of

home, staffing, occupancy levels, dependency levels, or staff psychological distress.
- However compared with the other two clusters, Cluster 1 (*restrictive*) had scores which indicated significantly higher work demands and role conflict, and significantly lower job satisfaction and a climate of lower effort.

8 The Views of Relatives

Although the study was principally focused on older people and their quality of life, relatives are important contributors to an older person's quality of life, and also can make important, and perhaps objective, judgements about quality. The Centre for Policy and Ageing (CPA) document *Fit for the Future* (Department of Health, 1999) cites the importance of continuing contact with relatives in the long-term care of older people. In this chapter, the views of relatives who were in close contact with the resident are examined regarding admission, their role in caring for the resident and quality of care in the homes.

Questionnaires were sent to relatives on three occasions, shortly after each of the three resident interviews. The relatives were not necessarily next of kin — the criterion was that they were to be the most likely to visit or keep in contact with the resident. In a few cases the recipient of the questionnaire was a close friend, and in one case a professional home carer continued a friendship with the resident after admission and was sent a questionnaire. The term 'relatives' is used here to refer to all the questionnaire respondents. Two forms of the questionnaire were produced. The 'time 1' version included sections which asked for information about the relative and his or her relationship to the resident, and about pre-admission decision making. These items were excluded from the versions sent on the follow-up occasions. An exception to this was that relatives who had not responded at time 1 were sent the full version of the questionnaire at time 2, thus providing a second opportunity to obtain the additional information. There were a few relatives who responded at time 2 having failed to respond at time 1.

Relatives' questionnaires were returned at time 1 in relation to 189 of the 308 cohort residents, giving a response rate of 61.36 per cent, which would usually be considered acceptable for a postal questionnaire. The personal and admission process data from a further 11 questionnaires received at time 2 was added to this where appropriate, so that some baseline relatives information is available on 200 of the 308 residents. The mean age of the 200 relatives was 58.4 years (std.dev. 12.7 years), the youngest being 26 and the oldest 90, and 63.3 per cent were female.

Table 8.1 shows the relationship between respondents to the questionnaire and the residents they visited. It can be seen that daughters were the largest group of respondents, although a significant number of sons also completed questionnaires. 'Other relatives' included cousins, nieces and nephews. Sixty-one per cent of the relatives had been the main carers of residents prior to admission. In the light of this it is not surprising to find that the majority lived quite near the home — 86 per cent lived within 30 minutes travelling time.

Table 8.1
Respondents to the relatives' questionnaire

	Number	Per cent
Wife	16	8.2
Husband	11	5.6
Daughter	81	41.3
Son	42	21.4
Grandchild	2	1
Sibling	10	5.1
Other relative	28	14.3
Friend/professional carer	6	3.1

The relatives were asked whether they, or the residents themselves, had visited the home prior to the resident's admission. Fewer than half of the residents had visited the home before they arrived to live in it. By contrast 83 per cent of the relatives had visited before the admission, demonstrating their significance in the choice of home and admission decisions generally. Asked about factors which influenced the choice of home, more relatives cited 'general good reputation' (48 per cent) and nearness to their (the relative's) home (47 per cent) than any other factors, although nearness to the resident's home and professional recommendations were also important. More than a quarter of the relatives mentioned that the home was already known, having been used, for example, for respite or day care.

For 68 per cent of the relatives information had been available to help them make the choice of home, although it is perhaps more noteworthy that this means nearly a third of them had received no information of any kind. Of those who received information, just under 70 per cent considered it to have been of good quality. The largest source of pre-admission information came from the homes themselves (for 30 per cent of all the responding relatives).

Other sources included: social services departments or social workers (27 per cent); other professional sources such as doctors, hospitals and health authorities (9 per cent) and friends (4.5 per cent). Given the role of social services departments in the assessment and admission process it is perhaps surprising to find that only 27 per cent of relatives had received from this source any information to help them make a decision between homes. Thirty-three of the people who did receive social services information thought it was good, while the other 20 described it as being 'fair' or 'poor'.

Questioned a short time after the admission, many of the relatives were very frequent, if not daily, visitors — indeed 93 per cent visited at least once a week. The vast majority (91 per cent) said they were always made to feel welcome when they visited the home. Most — though not quite all (73 per cent) — were offered tea or coffee when they visited and 15 per cent were offered meals if they visited at a mealtime. Eighty-three per cent said they enjoyed their visits but 25 people (14 per cent) did not and another six expressed mixed feelings. A number of those who did not enjoy their visits added notes to their questionnaires to explain that this was not because of a problem with the home, but because they found it distressing to see the resident in any home, or reduced to so ill or disabled a state.

They were asked how they spent their time while visiting. The almost universal activity was of course 'chatting with resident' — although this was not possible for some visitors who noted that communication was impossible. Over a third took residents out. Nearly a quarter carried out personal care tasks — some noted that staff would do these things but they or the resident preferred to do the cutting of nails or brushing of hair. A few visited at mealtimes in order to feed the resident — there were occasional comments that staff could not take the time necessary to spoon-feed properly. Perhaps because the admission had been recent a number of relatives dealt with business matters and delivered post. Ninety per cent took with them any items needed by the resident and quite a few spent time sorting clothes and taking items home for washing. That 28 per cent spent time talking to staff and discussing the resident's difficulties is perhaps also connected with the fact that the admission had been very recent. One relative reported that s/he was able to have a pre-booked lunch with the resident and that this made the visit more pleasurable. Moriarty and Webb (2000) reported that a substantial number of former carers continued to provide personal care after the older person they cared for had been admitted to a home. They suggested that the care homes in their study co-operated well with relatives who wished to continue with this level of involvement.

Relatives were asked some specific questions about the home, its staff, and the approach to residents generally. The experience of the majority (70 per cent) of the relatives at this early stage was that staff were always available to answer any questions they might have. Most of them (88 per cent) also observed that staff were nearly always or usually available to help residents. Only thirteen relatives thought that all the staff always 'talked down' to the residents. The majority (72 per cent) said that this never happened.

A number of other questions about home quality were asked specifically in relation to residents and these responses are set out in Table 8.2. In this table the percentage of relatives who responded positively to each of the questions is shown. It should be noted that these are all valid percentages, thus leaving out of the calculation those respondents who did not answer particular questions. Some of the questions clearly caused more difficulty than others and were often left unanswered. For each question the number of valid responses is given in the 'N' column: the lower this number the higher the number of relatives who left the question unanswered. There was, for instance, much more uncertainty (as well as more certainty of a negative response) about whether residents had enough to do than about whether they had a comfortable room. On the subject of activity, although two-thirds of respondents answered 'yes' as to whether their residents had enough to do in the home, just 56 per cent of respondents (n=93) thought they had enough things to do all or most of the time.

Relatives were given an opportunity to record any comments they wished to make about the homes, or about the care received by the residents, whether

Table 8.2
Quality questions: the experience of the visited resident

Question	% of relatives answering 'yes'	N= (max. possible = 189)
Do you think the staff have taken trouble to find out about (the resident's):		
background	82.7	156
difficulties	92.5	148
cultural/religious needs	76.2	126
interests	76.2	143
Do you think (the resident) is safe from:		
intruders	93.4	181
other residents	89.5	171
him/herself (accidents etc.)	90.2	173
Do you think (the resident) has:		
a homely and comfortable room	97.7	177
a pleasant lounge to sit in	97.3	183
a pleasant garden to sit in when fine	89.4	179
enough privacy	89.7	175
food he/she enjoys	92.4	171
enough to do	66.7	153

favourable or unfavourable. A number of them used this opportunity. Fifty-four people made comments about staff and 80 per cent of these were favourable — that staff were pleasant, friendly, caring, competent. This included three relatives who commented that the home had a good staff/resident ratio. The remaining eleven relatives who had criticisms to make were nearly all concerned with staff shortage and delays in residents receiving attention.

Comments about the building and accommodation were made by 22 people: 15 said that it was clean, comfortable and pleasant, five that it was dirty, shabby or smelly, and two criticised inadequate security. Only 14 relatives added specific comments on activity and social opportunities in the home: five thought they were good and varied; nine would have liked to see more, or better, opportunities.

Thirty-four other comments were made which were varied in nature, mainly relating to the physical environment of the home or the care received:

- life for resident would be better if the other residents were less disabled, mentally and better able to communicate / livelier (4 comments);
- the food is poor / meals too small / not enough spent on food (4);
- the food is good (2);
- care generally or specific services too expensive / local authority help with charges should be available (4);
- home very well and professionally managed (4);
- an institution managed for profit by people who do not care (1);
- residents not given enough baths (1);
- not enough wardrobe space (1);
- well equipped / modern (1);
- would prefer resident to be in a single room (1);
- would prefer resident to be in a shared room — is too isolated (1);
- toilet facilities poor (1);
- wheelchairs have foot rests missing (1);
- poor crockery; inadequate equipment for feeding disabled people (1);
- insufficient armchairs in lounge (1);
- resident should be allowed to keep some of pension money (1);
- clothes go missing / are damaged in the wash; hearing aids go missing (2);
- residents would benefit from more 'sign-posting' — to find way around home, giving day of week, etc. (1);
- staff put residents to bed too early (1);
- monthly financial statements should be provided for relatives (1).

Relatives were asked to give two separate ratings designed to measure their satisfaction or otherwise with the home and the care received by the resident. The first was a simple five-point scale ranging from 'very satisfied' to 'very dissatisfied' in response to the question 'Generally speaking, how satisfied are you with the cleanliness, appearance and comfort of the home overall?' The responses are illustrated in Figure 8.1 and reveal a very high level of satisfaction.

Figure 8.1
Relatives' satisfaction

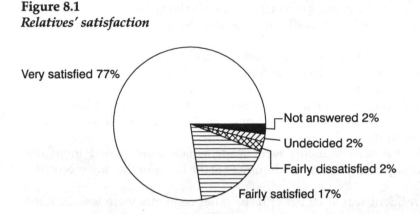

The other rating required relatives to choose one of three possible statements, expressed as follows: Please think about the care this home provides, taking into account anything at all which seems relevant to you. Please then decide which of the following statements best describes your views:

- I am very happy to see my relative living here. I feel completely reassured that the best possible care is being provided.
- I feel fairly happy about seeing my relative living here. I have some doubts about the home but I think it provides a reasonable quality of care.
- I am not happy about my relative living here. I think this home provides rather poor quality of care and if possible I would have chosen another one.

This question also elicited a high level of satisfaction, with almost three quarters of the relatives saying that they were very happy to see the resident living in the home and felt completely reassured that the best possible care was being provided.

It should be noted that, while the relatives appeared to be highly satisfied with the homes overall, a number of those who gave high satisfaction ratings had, earlier in the questionnaire, expressed some quite serious criticisms. It is possible that, in the difficult period around admission, some relatives' feelings of relief preclude expression of dissatisfaction even when specific shortcomings have been noted.

In summary

- Questionnaires were posted to relatives on three occasions. At time 1, 189 out of 308 were returned, giving a response rate of 61.4 per cent. Daughters made up the largest group of respondents although a significant proportion was received from sons.
- Although less than half of all residents had visited the homes prior to admission, 83 per cent of relatives did so. Relatives cited 'good reputation' (48 per cent) and 'nearness' (47 per cent) as factors which influenced choice of home.
- During their visits to the homes, the majority of relatives spent time 'chatting with the resident'. One-third of relatives took residents out and almost a quarter carried out personal tasks for the residents. A small number of relatives visited at mealtimes to assist with feeding.
- The vast majority of relatives thought that their resident had a comfortable room, a pleasant lounge or garden to sit in, enough privacy and good food. However, one-third of respondents answered 'no' when asked whether their resident had enough to do in the home.
- With regard to general cleanliness, appearance and comfort of the home, there was overall a very high level of satisfaction (77 per cent very satisfied). A question regarding quality of care received by the resident also elicited a high level of satisfaction with almost three-quarters of relatives very happy with the home, despite the fact that a number of specific criticisms were reported in some questionnaires.

9 Cognitive Impairment and Interviewability*

Any research or service evaluation involving questionnaires or interviewing of older people, particularly the very old or those living in care homes, has to take into account the likelihood that some potential subjects will be cognitively impaired and may be unable to understand or give appropriate answers to questions (Albert, 1998). When the presence or otherwise of cognitive impairment is the subject of investigation the question of whether the respondent can give accurate or meaningful responses does not arise. It becomes important when the questions are on any other subject, including symptoms, mood state or functional difficulties. It is certainly an issue for any study where the questions to which answers are sought concern life history, opinions and attitudes, quality of life evaluation or satisfaction with services. According to some authors, subjects with Alzheimer's Disease 'cannot comprehend questions or report on subjective states' (Albert, 1998) or, more extremely, they 'approach more closely the condition of animals than normal adult humans in their psychological capacities' (Buchanan and Brock, 1989).

Some large studies of older people and their care services have avoided direct interviewing altogether, preferring to concentrate on information from third-party informants and observation (for example, Booth, 1985, Albert et al., 1996). In direct interviewing it is common to exclude those deemed unable to participate, by using staff or other third-party views that potential subjects are

---

* With contextual alterations, the substance of this chapter was first published as 'Not knowing where I am doesn't mean I don't know what I like': cognitive impairment and quality of life responses in elderly people, Mozley, C. et al., *International Journal of Geriatric Psychiatry* (1999) 14, 776–783.

'(very) confused' (for example, Willcocks et al., 1987; Allen et al., 1992; Tulle-Winton, 1995; Myers and MacDonald, 1996). In a major study of residential homes carried out in Scotland, Bland et al. (1992) included interviews with residents of six homes. Six residents were randomly selected in each home but substitutions were made for residents deemed by a member of the home's staff to have dementia. Sometimes it is not entirely clear whether or how cognitively impaired subjects were excluded but the context makes it quite likely that they were (for example, Reed and Roskell-Payton, 1996). Some studies have used the Mini Mental State Examination (MMSE) (Folstein et al., 1975) as an interview screen but do not report the precise scoring threshold used. For example Reed and Gilleard (1995) interviewed 125 older people about their satisfaction with community nursing services and used a modified version of the MMSE to exclude those with moderate to severe dementia or confusion. Studies which have attempted this type of interview without any screening decision (for example Challis et al., 1997; 2002a) are rare.

This issue is important for social and health policy because of the emphasis in recent years on the need to involve users of services in the planning and evaluation of their care. There has been considerable research interest in those who care for relatives with dementia, both in their own right and as proxies to represent the views of older people themselves (Qureshi and Walker, 1989; Levin et al., 1994). However, the views of carers and family members, though important, are not a substitute for those of older service users and there is evidence that researchers are increasingly interested in finding ways of involving cognitively impaired people in research and evaluation (Downs, 1997).

The use in this study of the MMSE as a screen before further quality of life interviewing provided an opportunity to look at the relationship between MMSE score and interviewability. It was anticipated that there would be, in the study population, a number of respondents who would have difficulty with the Lancashire Quality of Life Profile–Residential (LQOLP-R). It was, therefore, decided that the MMSE would be used as a consistent basis for screening out those who were too cognitively impaired. It was originally planned to use 17/18 as the screening cut-off score, in line with many researchers who regard this as indicative of severe impairment (Tombaugh and McIntyre, 1992). During a small series of interviews done for preliminary testing and interviewer training it became clear that there were people with MMSE scores lower than 17 who were, nevertheless, able to answer at least some of the quality of life questions. Following this observation, and based on the clinical experience of one of the authors, the cut-off was reduced to 9/10.

Data from the first round of interviews were analysed to determine the extent to which the MMSE succeeded in providing solid grounds for sorting respondents into two groups — those who were, and those who were not interviewable on the subject of their quality of life. In this context 'interviewable' is defined as 'able to answer the majority of questions in the LQOLP-R and in doing so to give answers in which the interviewer has confidence'. This was quantified by counting two things — the proportion of answered questions and the number of interview sections (out of nine) for which the interviewer recorded confidence in the responses. This second step was necessary to deal with responses which were adequate if taken at face value, but probably affected by disordered thinking. For example, it is possible for a respondent to answer 'yes, very satisfied' in response to a series of questions about the home, its food, its comfort and services while interspersing these responses with comments which make it plain that she thinks she is living in her own mother's care.

Interviewers made these confidence ratings as the interview proceeded by using a three-point coding labelled *reliable / unreliable / mixed*. Nine interview sections were rated separately because respondents might be more interested in some subjects, or might improve or deteriorate as rapport developed or declined. The *mixed* rating acted as a buffer zone for occasions of doubt, such as when responses seemed repetitive and compliant. It is important to note that a conservative approach was taken to attaching the label of interviewer confidence, by excluding interview sections rated *mixed*. Interviews for which a clear majority — at least six of the nine sections — were rated *reliable* were classified as interviews with interviewer confidence. Since in almost all cases these were also interviews where the majority of questions had been answered, this binary interviewer confidence variable could be used as a summary to define whether a reasonably complete and reliable LQOLP-R interview was achieved and thus to quantify the condition of 'interviewability'. Inter-rater reliability for the interviewer confidence variable was tested for a series of 26 co-rated interviews (one person interviewing while another independently recorded a second set of responses and confidence ratings) and found to be high (K = 0.69, p < 0.001).

Of the 308 screened residents, 213 (69 per cent) scored 10 or more on the MMSE and a quality of life interview was attempted. Of these 213, 55 per cent scored at or below 17, the score often taken as the threshold for defining severe impairment (Tombaugh and McIntyre, 1992). There were some differences between the group of 213 quality of life respondents and the 95 who failed to reach a score of 10 on the MMSE (the 'above threshold' and 'below threshold' groups). The two groups were not significantly different in age but were different in gender and level of care. The screened cohort of 308 residents was two-thirds female (96 men, 212 women). There were 60.4 per cent of the men and 73.1 per cent of the women who scored above the 9/10 threshold and became quality of life interview respondents ($\chi^2(1) = 4.99$, p = 0.025). Of the 95 below threshold exclusions from further interview 69 (67 per cent) were in nursing, as opposed to residential homes ($\chi^2(1) = 13.64$, p < 0.001).

MMSE sub-scores for the seven domains of orientation to time, orientation to place, language, attention, visual construction, registration and recall were examined in both groups. As Table 9.1 illustrates, respondents who achieved scores of 10 or over did so in various ways. The language domain, with its possible maximum score of 8, was an important component of an above threshold score for many people; indeed, no-one achieved a total score of 10 or more with a zero score for language. However the above threshold scorers were not in this position simply because 8 points were available for language — more than a third of them had language scores of 4 or less. Of the above threshold scorers (with whom quality of life interviews were attempted), some scored zero for orientation to time (10.7 per cent) and place (9.3 per cent), while complete failure was recorded by as many as 64.1 per cent of them for the visual construction task and 66.2 per cent for recall. Comparison of the proportion of the above threshold and below threshold groups scoring at or above the mid-point score for each domain suggests that many people were able to score 2 or 3

Table 9.1
Respondents above and below the MMSE 9/10 threshold and the seven MMSE domains (all screened respondents: n=308)

MMSE domain (possible maximum domain score)	% respondents with MMSE < 10 who scored 0 for this domain	% respondents with MMSE > 10 who scored 0 for this domain	% respondents with MMSE < 10 and score for this domain at or above mid point	% respondents with MMSE >10 and score for this domain at or above mid point
Orientation to time (max. score 5)	76.8 (n=63)	10.7 (n=23)	1.1 (n=1)	49.1 (n=105)
Orientation to place (5)	58.8 (n=47)	9.3 (n=20)	5.4 (n=5)	63 (n=136)
Language (8)	35.1 (n=27)	0	1.1 (n=1)	57.4 (n=124)
Attention (5)	46.6 (n=34)	4.3 (n=9)	1.1 (n=1)	63.9 (n=138)
Visual construction (1)	90.3 (n=65)	64.1 (n=134)	9.7 (n=7)	35.9 (n=75)
Registration (3)	27 (n=20)	1.4 (n=3)	44.6 (n=41)	92.6 (n=200)
Recall (3)	95.9 (n=71)	66.2 (n=141)	1.1 (n=1)	15.7 (n=34)

(out of 3) for registration — repeating three words — while being unable to accumulate more than 7 or 8 points from the remainder of the test. Conversely only 15.7 per cent of the above threshold scorers were at or above the mid-point for the recall test — the majority of people had difficulty with this, whether or not they were able to accumulate 10 points in other ways.

There was a significant correlation between the number of 'interviewer confidence' interview sections (between zero and nine) and MMSE score ($r = 0.45$, $p <0.001$), thus the higher the MMSE score, the greater the degree of 'interviewer confidence'. The number of unanswered questions was inversely correlated with MMSE score ($r = -0.27$, $p <0.001$). Depression, measured by the GDS-15, had no effect on the association between interviewer confidence and MMSE score. Table 9.2 illustrates the fact that the percentage of interviewable respondents rose steadily with MMSE scores.

However, a number of residents were interviewable with the LQOLP-R despite having MMSE scores at the lower end of the range. With a threshold of MMSE 10, 77.5 per cent of the interviews were achieved satisfactorily. If the threshold had been 15 and over this proportion would have been very nearly 90 per cent — but it is not until the MMSE score of 26 and over is taken as the threshold that 100 per cent interviewability is achieved. The figure of 77.5 per cent at 10 or over is sufficiently large to encourage speculation that some respondents with even lower scores may have been interviewable.

Table 9.2
MMSE score and 'interviewability'

Selecting interviewees with MMSE scores of:	Percentage interviewable
10 and above	77.5 (n=213)
11 and above	81.3 (n=192)
12 and above	85.5 (n=173)
13 and above	87 (n=161)
14 and above	88 (n=150)
15 and above	89.8 (n=137)
16 and above	91.1 (n=124)
17 and above	93.6 (n=110)
18 and above	94.8 (n=97)
19 and above	96.4 (n=83)
20 and above	96.2 (n=78)
21 and above	95.7 (n=69)
22 and above	94.9 (n=59)
23 and above	95.7 (n=47)
24 and above	97 (n=33)
25 and above	96 (n=25)
26 and above	100 (n=18)

Because each of the nine interview sections was separately rated, it was possible to investigate whether interviewer confidence was attached to some interview sections more than to others. This was not found to be the case. For each section there was interviewer confidence in approximately 80 per cent of the interviews. In relation to questions about satisfaction with current living situation, arguably the most relevant section to the experience of being in a care home, the figure was 80.4 per cent.

To investigate whether greater cognitive impairment produced systematic differences in patterns of responses to the LQOLP-R questions, respondents scoring above and below MMSE 17/18 were compared using the 12-item Living Situation Scale. Internal consistency of the scale was similar in both groups (Cronbach's α = 0.91 and 0.82).

The data were then examined to see whether skills in some of the MMSE domains were particularly associated with interviewability. Table 9.3 shows that some domain scores more strongly associated with interviewability than others. The visual construction and registration tests were unhelpful — there was no statistically significant difference between the interviewable and non-interviewable respondents. All the other domains showed statistically significant differences between the two groups. However, *of the interviewable respondents*, low scores were obtained by 44 per cent for orientation to time and 81.2 per cent for recall. Thus inability to give the correct day, date or time did not necessarily render the person uninterviewable — nor did difficulty in recalling three words recently heard. The differences between the interviewable and non-interviewable groups in the three domains of attention, orientation to place and language were considerable and various

Table 9.3
MMSE domain differences between interviewable and non-interviewable respondents (all with MMSE scores 10 and above: n=213)

MMSE domain (possible maximum domain score)	% non-interviewable respondents with score for this domain below mid-point	% interviewable respondents with score for this domain below mid-point	χ^2 value (df = 1); two tailed significance
Orientation to time (maximum score 5)	72.9	44.2	12.231 p < 0.001
Orientation to place (5)	70.8	26.7	31.251 p < 0.001
Language (8)	58.3	37	6.977 p = 0.008
Attention (5)	60.4	28.5	16.520 p < 0.001
Visual construction (1)	71.7	61.3	ns
Registration (3)	6.3	7.9	ns
Recall (3)	93.8	81.2	4.357 p = 0.037

combinations of these domain scores were examined to see whether they performed better as an interviewability screen than the MMSE taken as a whole. Based on this sample of MMSE 10+ scorers, of those respondents who failed to score at least 2 for orientation to place *or* at least 3 for language *or* at least 2 for attention, none were interviewable. Successful quality of life interviews were achieved with 77.8 per cent of those who met at least one of those three criteria.

The staff informant assessments made using the Crichton Royal Confusion Sub-scale and the HONOS-65+ were examined in relation to interviewability. All were significantly correlated at the 0.001 level. As might be expected the correlation coefficient of the two staff informant assessments was high (Spearman's rho = 0.84) with lower coefficients between the Confusion Sub-scale and MMSE (−.0.55) and between HONOS 65 + rating and MMSE (-0.49). Correlations between interviewability and both staff assessment measures were similar (approx. −0.4 in both cases). Both staff assessment measures have conventional cut-points used to describe different levels of impairment. Staff were not asked the direct question 'is this person interviewable?' (with hindsight, this should have been asked). In the absence of this information the cut-points were used as proxies for staff judgements. This attempt to discriminate between interviewable and non-interviewable respondents on the basis of staff ratings did not prove particularly successful. Eighty-four of the respondents whose MMSE scores were above the 9/10 threshold scored 4 and over on the Confusion Sub-scale and would thus be regarded as moderately or severely confused in terms of this instrument. Of those 84 respondents 60.7 per cent were interviewable. Of the 11 respondents who scored 7 or more on the Confusion Sub-scale (i.e. at the 'severe confusion' level), six were interviewable. Using the HONOS-65+, 21 respondents who scored above the MMSE 9/10 threshold were classified as moderately or severely cognitively impaired and 13, or 61.9 per cent were interviewable. Thus, if these criteria had been used to decide who to include for LQOLP-R interview, large numbers of potential respondents would have been excluded.

For the purposes of this analysis the study had some methodological limitations. First, the decision to operate an MMSE screening threshold of 9/10 was taken on the basis of clinical judgement. Although the intention was to set it low enough to ensure maximum inclusion in quality of life interviewing, this has had the result of leaving unanswered questions about the interviewability of people with lower scores. Second, the interviewer confidence ratings were made by interviewers who had previously administered the MMSE, so the two measures cannot be treated as independent. Very poor scores on attention items or the fact that, while sitting in Manchester, the respondent thought himself in Birmingham would have had some influence on the subsequent confidence rating decision. Third, the study involved a cohort of people very recently admitted to care homes and it is possible that response patterns —

particularly in relation to orientation questions — may have been affected by this.

Nevertheless, the data point to some noteworthy conclusions. It is clear that many of those who attempted the LQOLP-R were cognitively impaired to a significant degree, with more than half of them scoring at or below 17 on the MMSE. Nevertheless, more than three-quarters of them were interviewable. That is, they were able to answer the majority of questions in the LQOLP-R and, in doing so, to give answers in which the interviewer had confidence. This percentage is probably higher than many people would expect to find in a very old population of care home residents and in the presence of this degree of cognitive impairment. If the MMSE cut-point of 17/18 had been chosen, the study would have obtained satisfactory quality of life interviews from 92 respondents instead of 165 — and yet this threshold is commonly taken to indicate severe impairment.

The objection might be made that opinions expressed by the more impaired respondents had no real meaning; that interviewers were fooled by a well pre-served social facade unsupported by coherent thought processes. However, all the interviewers were trained professionals with previous experience of older people with dementia and other mental health problems. On occasions of doubt they used the *mixed* confidence rating which was not included when calculating interviewability. It might also be thought that credence cannot be given to anything said by someone who does not, for example, know what year it is or where he is: that, in itself, failure to answer this type of question negates the value of further discussion. To a limited degree the findings of this study support this view, in that interviewability was significantly associated with orientation to place and attention. However some interviewable respon-dents failed key individual items. Sixty-three did not know the day of the week and 30 could not name the town they were in. These failures did not make further discussion pointless, because they often occurred in respondents who showed skill in other items. Of those who did not know the day of the week, 30 per cent scored full marks for spelling 'world' backwards and 57 per cent could write a complete sentence. Of those who did not know what town they were in, 25 per cent scored full marks for 'world' and 55 per cent wrote the sentence.

This serves merely as a reminder that cognitive impairment is a complex phenomenon and that some components of cognitive functioning are more essential to specific real life activities than others. It is probably inappropriate to assume incapacity to answer quality of life questions from inability to give the correct date, copy a diagram, write a sentence, or recall three unconnected and irrelevant words recently heard. On the other hand, the data support the view that a minimum level of orientation to place, language skill and attention are essential for interviewability and, in combination, these three domains appear to offer a way of isolating the cognitive skills required for successful quality of life interviewing. This conclusion is particularly important when decisions are made regarding the use of measures of service quality such as satisfaction (Cm 4169, 1998), and who should complete them.

In summary

The MMSE was designed as a clinical tool in order to probe all the various areas in which cognitive skills may have been lost. It has become well established in a research context although the requirements and attributes of a research instrument are not necessarily the same as those of a standardised clinical interview schedule. The MMSE, the Crichton Royal Confusion Sub-scale and the cognitive impairment assessment made in the HONOS-65+ all have the objective of indicating the presence of cognitive impairment — not the presence of interviewability. To attempt to use these clinicometric instruments to determine interviewability for another purpose, whatever it is, is probably mistaken. This study demonstrates that the MMSE cut-off of 17/18 commonly used to indicate severe impairment is a poor guide to quality of life interviewability. It has also been shown that some of the MMSE domains predict this better than others. Whether it is better to rely on these specific domains for future attempts to screen interviewable subjects will only be answered by further research involving interviewing across the full range of MMSE scores.

These findings do, however, suggest that it is possible to use direct rather than informant-based research methods with a higher proportion of older people than might be assumed — even in the presence of significant cognitive deficits. The essential requirements for interviewability appear to be a minimum level of orientation to place, attention and language skill. If many such people are indeed capable of expressing a meaningful opinion on the circumstances of their lives and the nature of the care and services they receive, this raises questions about the basis on which exclusions from research of this kind are made. Thus, studies should attempt to include as many subjects as possible using direct interview methods and report clear criteria for any exclusions. Finally, it is perhaps inadvisable to operate a screening procedure for interviewability based either on the full MMSE or on the judgements of third parties.

10 Recognition and Assessment of Depression

Staff recognition of depression*

A number of community and hospital based studies have investigated the ability of health care professionals to recognise depression, and report that under-diagnosis and inadequate treatment are common (Koenig et al., 1988; Rapp et al., 1988; Bowers et al., 1990; Pond et al., 1990; Heston et al., 1992; Shah and De, 1998). Bowers et al. (1990) reported that 80 per cent of cases of depression were not recognised by general practitioners. Jackson and Baldwin (1993) investigated the depression detection rates of nurses working in acute admission wards for older people. They were asked to make an assessment using a four-point scale: 'definitely not depressed', 'probably not depressed', 'probably depressed' and 'definitely depressed'. The ratings were compared with a researcher's rating of depression using the Geriatric Mental State Schedule (GMSS) (Copeland et al., 1976). When the responses were collapsed into 'depressed' and 'not depressed' the depression recognition rate of the nurses studied was only 38 per cent. This suggests that the nurses were missing important cues about symptoms of depression.

In residential homes, Schneider et al. (1997a) found that, of 77 residents classified as depressed using the Brief Assessment Schedule (BAS) (Mann et al., 1984), only 13 had been identified as such by key workers. Within a larger study Ames (1990) assessed the ability of residential home managers to recognise residents as depressed. Of 93 residents assessed as depressed (again

---

* With contextual alterations, the substance of this section was first published as 'Recognition of depression by staff in nursing and residential homes', in Bagley, H. et al., *Journal of Clinical Nursing* (2000) 9, 445–450.

using the BAS) they judged 35 'not depressed', 33 'mildly depressed', 16 'moderately' and seven 'severely' depressed. The authors concluded that managers used a higher threshold than the BAS for identifying depression.

Several factors have been suggested for the 'non-recognition' of depression in older people. A number of putative depressive symptoms may be present due to disorders other than depression, for example poor appetite, sleep problems and memory loss. Depressive symptoms can also be perceived as an understandable reaction to the loss, bereavement, ill-health and loss of social status which often accompanies ageing. As well as reinforcing negative attitudes to ageing, such viewpoints may impair recognition of significant and treatable mood changes.

Older people entering long-term care facilities face major adjustment challenges and are particularly vulnerable to mental health problems (Murphy, 1982; Mikhail, 1992; Manion and Rantz, 1995). The first few weeks in a care home have been described as the 'disorganisation' phase (Brooke, 1989), during which residents may experience feelings of abandonment, vulnerability and displacement. The circumstances of admission may have been very stressful and many residents enter homes at a point of crisis, for example, following sudden deterioration in health (Chenitz, 1983; Challis and Davies, 1986; Willcocks et al., 1987). At this potentially chaotic time in an older person's life it is crucial that staff are particularly sensitive to the risk of mental health problems.

The resident/care staff relationship provides an opportunity for recognising symptoms of depression and referring sufferers for further assessment and treatment if required. While care staff are not responsible for 'diagnosing', as daily providers of care it is important for them to have the ability both to recognise symptoms of depression and make appropriate referrals. Blanchard et al. (1995) introduced a variety of (primary care) nurse led interventions such as behavioural therapy, new assessment procedures and medication trials with a community sample of depressed older people. A significant three-month improvement in GMSS rated depression was found in the intervention group compared with a control group receiving usual GP care. Although this study does not directly address the issue of depression recognition, it demonstrates that once depression is recognised, nurse led interventions may have some success in management and treatment of depression. It is also known that recognition of common mental disorders results in improved outcome, even in the absence of intervention (Goldberg and Huxley, 1992).

The data collected for this study at 'time 1' were analysed to investigate:

- the ability of care staff to recognise depression in newly admitted residents of nursing and residential homes;
- whether qualified nursing staff were more likely to recognise depression than care staff with no formal training;

- the level of training in psychological care received by staff within residential and nursing homes.

The informant interviews which provide the basis of the assessment of staff depression recognition were carried out after the Geriatric Depression Scale interviews with a member of staff who had prior knowledge of the resident. These were staff who had care responsibilities for the resident and it would be reasonable to expect them to be made aware of any significant identified health problems.

The likelihood of bias due to staff giving socially desirable responses to the depression question was minimised by the fact that it was included in an interview about a range of residents' problems including activities of daily living, illnesses and disabilities. The question formed part of the Health of the Nation Outcome Scale for older people (HONOS-65+) (Burns et al., 1999), an informant rated 12-item score, and took the form: 'Has [name of resident] had any problems with depressive symptoms during the past week?' The categories and ratings used to record the informant's response are set out in Table 10.1.

Table 10.1
HONOS-65+ depression rating categories

0	No problems associated with depression during the period rated
1	Gloomy, minor changes in mood only
2	Mild but definite depression on subjective and/or objective measures (e.g. loss of interest and/or pleasure, lack of energy, loss of self esteem, feelings of guilt)
3	Moderate depression on subjective and/or objective grounds (depressive symptoms more marked)
4	Severe depression on subjective and/or objective grounds (e.g. profound loss of interest and/or pleasure with ideas of guilt or worthlessness)

The data were dichotomised in order that a depressed/not depressed staff rating could be developed from the original 5-point HONOS-65+ scale. The cut-point for depressed/not depressed was empirically determined. Staff used the 'gloomy' category regularly compared to the 'mild but definite depression category' or any other 'definite depression' ratings. Consequently two methods of examining the data were used when comparing the staff rating with the case/non-case rating of depression from the GDS-15 assessment. Subsequent analysis is, therefore, based on two methods. The first method involved classifying 'no problems with depression' versus anything from 'gloomy' to severe depression (i.e. ratings of 0 compared with ratings of 1, 2, 3, or 4). The second method classified 'no problems' and 'gloomy' together versus anything from mild to severe depression (i.e. ratings of 0 or 1 compared with ratings of 2, 3 or

4). This rating assumes that the 'gloomy' symptoms recognised by the staff member were not regarded as depressive symptoms, merely minor changes in mood.

There were 248 residents with valid GDS-15 scores at time 1. Three of these residents were excluded from this analysis because staff members had been unable to supply information relating to the question on depression. Of the remaining 245 residents, 107 (43.7 per cent) were classed as depressed on the GDS-15 using the 5/6 cut-point. The mean GDS-15 score for interviewed residents was 5.3 (std.dev. 3.2). There were no statistically significant differences between GDS-15 scores for residents in nursing or residential homes. The informant question on depression was completed by 98 nurses and 147 'other' care staff.

When HONOS-65+ ratings of 1 or higher (i.e. gloomy or worse) were viewed as recognition of depression, staff detected only 27.1 per cent (n=29) of those identified as 'cases' using the GDS-15. When 'gloomy' was not included as a depression rating the recognition rate fell to 15 per cent (n=16). When 'gloomy' was included with the more severe depression categories, qualified nurses identified just over a third (36.4 per cent) of GDS-15 'cases'. When the second method was used (i.e. when scores of 2 or higher were viewed as recognition of depression) only 20.5 per cent of cases were recognised by qualified nurses. Recognition rates of other care staff were similar (20.6 per cent and 11.1 per cent for the first and second method respectively). There were no significant differences in recognition rates between nursing and other care staff. Thus the nursing and care staff in this study demonstrated a low rate of recognition of depression in newly admitted residents. In this there was essentially no difference between qualified nursing staff and unqualified care staff.

Training

The information on staff training in the psychological care of residents came from the postal questionnaire completed by 332 care and nursing staff (see Chapter 6). Of the 332 staff questionnaire respondents only 26 (7.8 per cent) had received any training in 'psychological or psychiatric' care while employed in their current place of employment. On further examination, however, in only six cases (1.8 per cent) did the responses suggest any possibility of training in depression — indeed in only one case was the word depression actually used. The other respondents appear to have attended more general training courses on 'mental health' which might be assumed to contain an element of training on depression. The mean period of time in employment in the current care facility was 4.2 years (std.dev. = 2.9 years).

Training of staff to recognise depression was, therefore, virtually non-existent in the homes studied. There are reasons for treating the staff training data with some caution. First, information about previous training and qualifications was obtained, but it is impossible to extract from this precise and comparable data on subject content. For this reason the data used here concern only the *amount* and *type* of in-service training received in the current place of employment. It could be argued that this has the effect of under-estimating the training of staff, but since the mean employment time in the present workplace was over four years it seems reasonable to suggest that even previously trained staff should have received some 'updating' in that time. Second, it is possible that a small number of the senior care staff informants were qualified nurses who had chosen to work in residential homes. If so, this would tend to reduce the differences between the two groups compared in the analysis. However the depression recognition rates were so low for qualified nurses that this factor is unlikely to have been significant. Finally, staff training data were not collected at the time of the informant interview, making it impossible to relate depression recognition by an individual staff member to that person's training history. Again, since the level of relevant training in the staff population was so low it would be difficult to argue that the findings were biased as a result.

This analysis illustrates a general failure of nursing and residential staff to recognise depression in homes (as measured by GDS-15). Staff appeared to under-estimate residents' emotional needs, classifying a large number of depressed individuals as having either no depressive symptoms or only minor mood changes ('gloominess'). Moreover, this was very shortly after admission, when staff might have been expected to be particularly alert to depressive symptoms.

Since nurse training includes psychological care of patients it might be assumed that qualified nurses would be more likely than other carers to recognise depressive symptoms. This was not the case in this study. The nurses failed to recognise any problems with depressive symptoms in two-thirds of cases and their rates of recognition were comparable with those of staff without formal nurse training. It therefore appears that the training nurses receive does not equip them to recognise depressive symptoms. This is a significant finding in light of the view of the Royal College of Nursing (RCN) that there are specific skills provided and values introduced by the presence of a qualified nurse in giving long-term care in nursing and residential homes. In a publication about the role of the nurse in this context the RCN emphasises the specific value of qualified nurses as 'skilled practitioners' in conducting assessments with older patients. It suggests that nurses note patients' responses and identify problems such as withdrawal or depression while talking to them (Royal College of Nursing, 1996).

The finding that under 2 per cent of staff respondents had received training relevant to the psychological care of residents suggests that this area was not seen as a priority in the homes studied. With increasing discussion of expanding the role of nurses into the provision of psychological interventions (Mead et al., 1997) this highlights a more fundamental training need — that of increasing the ability of staff appropriately to assess the psychological needs of clients. Until this ability is demonstrated, there seems to be limited value in progressing into the area of nursing interventions. Further investigation of the reasons for failure to recognise depression and increased understanding of professional knowledge and attitudes in relation to ageing and depression might help shape appropriate training for staff, improving both professional performance and the quality of life of those in their care.

A new version of the Geriatric Depression Scale*

Although the 30-item GDS has been shown to be effective in distinguishing between depressed and non-depressed older people (Yesavage, 1983), findings on the scale's use with cognitively impaired people are somewhat conflicting. Burke et al. (1992) reported that it performed as well with cognitively impaired individuals as with those without such difficulties. Parmalee et al. (1989) found no differences in its reliability and validity between cognitively impaired and unimpaired nursing home residents. However, an American study of 169 residents newly admitted to long-term care facilities found that it was a better screening instrument for depression in cognitively intact people (Kafonek et al., 1989).

The briefer GDS-15, which was used in this study, was designed to be easier for cognitively impaired people to complete (Sheikh and Yesavage, 1986). In research conducted in a nursing home setting (Gerety et al., 1994), the GDS-30 and the GDS-15 were found to be equally appropriate for use with people without severe dementia. Attempts have been made to create even shorter versions of the Geriatric Depression Scale. The GDS-10 and GDS-4 have been found acceptable to respondents in general practice settings (D'Ath et al., 1994) and in an acute geriatric hospital (Shah et al., 1997). Analysis of the large series of interviews carried out for this study, however, showed inadequate levels of consistency between the 15-, 10- and 4-item versions, as described in Chapter 5. It will be recalled that, using recommended cut-points 'caseness' rates of 44.8 per cent, 55.6 per cent and 67.3 per cent were identified in the same sample using the 15-, 4- and 10-item versions respectively.

---

*   With contextual alterations, the substance of this section was first published as 'A new version of the Geriatric Depression Scale for nursing and residential home populations: the Geriatric Depression Scale (Residential) (GDS-12R), Sutcliffe, C. et al., *International Psychogeriatrics* (2000) 12, 2, 173–181.

This section reports the development of the GDS-12R, a screening measure appropriate for use with older people in nursing and residential care. Data from all the interviews carried out for this study at times 1, 2, and 3, were used to investigate the internal reliability of the GDS-15, resulting in the exclusion of items which were poor identifiers of depression in this particular population.

It will be recalled that all residents were given a screener interview which included the MMSE and the GDS-15, the latter administered by the interviewer rather than as a self completed questionnaire because many residents had visual and other disabilities. Those scoring 10 or more on the MMSE also completed an adapted version of the Lancashire Quality of Life Profile (LQOLP-R). It is worth noting that most residents who scored 10 or more on the MMSE were capable of understanding and completing most of the quality of life questionnaire (see Chapter 9). The latter incorporated the Affect Balance Scale (ABS) (Bradburn, 1969), a subjective measure of psychological well-being with ten items in two subscales, relating to 'positive' and 'negative' affect. Although not developed for older people specifically, it has been found to be applicable to this population and to have acceptable levels of validity and reliability.

The development of the GDS-12R

During interviewing, researchers reported problems with some of the GDS-15 items. The circumstances in which many of the residents found themselves meant that they considered some questions irrelevant or ambiguous. For example, when asked, 'Do you prefer staying in rather than going out and doing new things?', many residents said they simply could not go out (indeed some were bed-bound). Some misunderstood the meaning of the item, 'Do you think that most people are better off than you are?', taking it as a reference to their financial situation following admission to the home.

One difficulty of this study was that, in the absence of a clinical diagnosis of depression, it was necessary to find another indicator of depression with which to compare the GDS-15 items for validity. Although not perfect, a single item was selected from the Affect Balance Scale, 'During the past month, did you ever feel depressed or very unhappy?'. This seemed appropriate because it was a direct question about *current or recent mood* and avoided reference to somatic symptoms of depression. The item was scored as dichotomous.

Subsequently, responses to each GDS-15 item were examined in detail to see if a shorter, more appropriate instrument would increase the reliability and validity of the scale. Analyses were carried out that compared each GDS-15 item response with the ABS item: 'During the past month, did you ever feel depressed or very unhappy?'. Crosstabulating the scores from each GDS-15 item with the responses to the latter indicated that all the GDS-15 items, apart from three, two of which are mentioned above, were significantly associated. The three GDS items not significantly associated with the ABS item were:

Do you prefer staying in, rather than going out and doing new things?
Do you feel that you have more problems with memory than most?
Do you think that most people are better off than you are?

That is, residents answering 'Yes' to the ABS item were more likely to give 'depressed' responses to the remaining twelve GDS items (see Table 10.2). This supported the decision to omit these three items from the scale for future analyses. Additionally using Cronbach α as a measure of internal reliability, it was found that omitting these three GDS-15 items increased α from 0.76 to 0.81. Internal reliability for the GDS-12R was then calculated for each of the three data collection periods: admission, five months and nine months. The alpha values were 0.805 (n=248), 0.848 (n=160), 0.812 (n=122) respectively. Although it could be argued that the three values are not independent, drawn as they were from the same sample, the fact that they are all high (all above 0.8) increases faith in the robustness of the shorter scale.

The cut points for the two versions of the GDS are given in Table 10.3 and Table 10.4. It is noticeable that using the ABS item as a comparison, the GDS-

Table 10.2
GDS-15 items — Affect Balance Scale single item

GDS-15 item	Affect Balance Scale item p values*	Valid N
Basic satisfaction	< 0.001	174
Dropped activities	0.014	178
Feels life empty	< 0.001	176
Often bored	< 0.001	178
In good spirits	0.004	177
Afraid something bad will happen	< 0.001	172
Feels happy	< 0.001	176
Often feels helpless	< 0.001	176
Prefers to stay in	0.217	172
More problems with memory than most	1.000	174
Wonderful to be alive	0.015	168
Feels worthless	< 0.001	174
Full of energy	0.006	176
Feels situation is hopeless	< 0.001	172
Most people better off than self	0.175	165

Note: * Fisher's Exact Test.

12R gives higher levels of specificity and sensitivity for this sample when compared with the corresponding cut points of the GDS-15. The figures in Table 10.4 suggest a cut point of 4/5 would be useful for research purposes. This gives the optimum values for both sensitivity and specificity and may be preferable where the 'purity' of the sample is important. However, it could also be envisaged that practitioners are more interested in increasing the

Table 10.3
Cut points for the GDS-15

Cut point of the GDS-15	Sensitivity %	Specificity %
0/1	96.4	6.4
1/2	95.2	21.3
2/3	88.1	34.0
3/4	83.3	52.1
4/5	**78.6**	**67.0**
5/6	69.0	76.6
6/7	60.7	85.1
7/8	48.8	91.5
8/9	36.9	94.7
9/10	25.0	97.9
10/11	15.5	100
11/12	8.3	100
12/13	2.4	100
13/14	2.4	100
14/15	0	100

Table 10.4
Cut points for the GDS-12R

Cut point of the GDS-12R	Sensitivity %	Specificity %
0/1	95.2	10.6
1/2	95.2	30.9
2/3	83.3	50.0
3/4	**78.6**	**69.1**
4/5	**72.6**	**76.6**
5/6	57.1	86.2
6/7	46.6	93.6
7/8	38.1	95.7
8/9	22.6	98.9
9/10	13.1	100
10/11	1.2	100
11/12	0	100

proportion of depressed people who are detected and are not so concerned with the specificity. In that situation a cut point of 3/4 would be more useful. This illustrates the importance of the 'trade off' between sensitivity (the proportion of true positives identified) and specificity (the proportion of true negatives identified) (Bowns et al., 1991).

Assessing depression in older people with cognitive impairment

A number of previous studies which used the GDS chose to exclude subjects with low MMSE scores. For example, Gerety et al. (1994) only included those with MMSE scores of 15 or above; McCrea et al. (1994) used a score of 21 as the criterion for inclusion. In contrast, for the current study all newly admitted residents were approached regardless of cognitive state. In fact 152 residents who were able to complete the GDS-15 scored below 18 on the MMSE. More importantly, there was no significant difference in internal reliability for the GDS-12R between those with MMSE scores above and below the MMSE cut-point of 17/18 commonly used to distinguish those with severe cognitive impairment. The alpha score for subjects scoring below the cut point of 18 was 0.80 indicating high internal reliability. Even for those with MMSE scores below 10 as used as a cut-point for this study, the alpha score was 0.78.

The GDS-15 has been used in preference to other measures of depression because it relies less on somatic symptoms of depression that may be exhibited by older non-depressed people. However, although the GDS-15 was designed for older people, it may not be entirely suitable for use with a very elderly population of care home residents. The analyses of the individual items of the GDS-15 concluded that internal reliability was highest when three items were removed. These were some of the items which had seemed problematic in the context of residential care. The answers to the three omitted items were not always a reflection of depressed mood but of the circumstances surrounding recent admission to long-term care and may have led to residents reaching the threshold score for 'depressed mood' without actually being depressed. The value of creating a new measure GDS-12R lies in the fact that it actually omits items which tend to mislead or confuse respondents who are answering from a different perspective, and results in greater accuracy of information. Furthermore, internal reliability on the GDS-12R remained high for residents who scored below the MMSE cut-points indicating moderate or severe cognitive impairment suggesting that the GDS-12R can be just as effective when used with older people who are cognitively impaired as with those who have little or no impairment.

The 12-item 'Residential' version of the Geriatric Depression Scale (the GDS-12R) shown in Box 10.1 appears to be a more suitable and reliable measure for use with older people in long-stay care homes including those with cognitive impairment, by removing less appropriate or ambiguous items from the

---

Box 10.1
GDS-12R questions

Are you basically satisfied with your life?
Have you dropped many of your activities and interests?
Do you feel that your life is empty?
Do you often get bored?
Are you in good spirits most of the time?
Are you afraid that something bad is going to happen to you?
Do you feel happy most of the time?
Do you often feel helpless?
Do you think it is wonderful to be alive now?
Do you feel pretty worthless the way you are now?
Do you feel full of energy?
Do you feel that your situation is hopeless?

GDS-15. In view of this, all subsequent statistical analyses have been undertaken using data derived from the 12-item GDS, rather than the GDS-15.

In summary

There are two important themes which emerge from this chapter. First, there was a very low level of recognition of depression (as measured by the HONOS-65+) by all grades of staff working in the homes. Furthermore, it appeared that the trained nursing staff in the homes were not significantly better than untrained staff in recognising depression. Secondly, the use of the GDS, a standard measure for assessing older people with regard to depression, did not appear to be fully appropriate in the context of a care home. Consequently, a new, shorter version of the GDS (GDS-12R) was created which was specific to the care home context.

Both of these findings are relevant in the light of recent policy changes in the care of older people arising from the *National Service Framework for Older People* (Department of Health, 2001b), in particular the specific guidance arising from the Single Assessment Process (SAP) in England (Department of Health, 2002a). The main focus of the Single Assessment Process Guidance, as in much of the development of assessment over the last decade, has been upon community based assessments. However, the case for more systematic assessment procedures in care homes is made more strongly by the evidence of poor detection rates for depression, irrespective of the occupational background of staff. There is considerable value too in a care home context specific tool for the assessment of depression, which could be used as part of the SAP (Department of Health, 2002a) or as part of the assessment required in standards 3 and 7 of the Care Standards for Residential Homes (Department of Health, 2001a).

11 The Outcomes of Care

In this chapter the study data are explored in various ways that begin to make use of their longitudinal characteristics. First, the extent to which some key variables changed over the period of the study is examined, to investigate whether the health status and quality of life indicators show improvement or deterioration over nine months of care home residence. For obvious reasons this analysis is based only on data for those residents who were alive throughout the nine-month study period.

Second, influences on survival are sought in the individual characteristics of residents and in characteristics of the care environment. Comparisons are made between three 'survival groups' — those who died in the first five months, those who died between five and nine months after admission and those who were alive at the end of the study. Data augmented by further survival follow-up data collected about a year after the end of the study are then used for Cox proportional hazards regression analysis (Cox and Oaks, 1984), to identify factors that made a significant contribution to the likelihood of survival.

Finally, multivariate techniques (both linear and logistic regression) are used to investigate the study's primary question — whether aspects of the care environment had a significant influence on the key resident outcomes at nine months post admission.

Changes in key variables for residents alive throughout the study

Of the original cohort of 308, 188 people were known to be alive after nine months. Of these, interviews were attempted with 188 at time 1, 184 at time 2 and 168 at time 3. However, some residents failed to complete particular scales and sample sizes for some variables are, therefore, lower than these numbers.

Depression

Data on changes in the GDS-12R scores from time 1 to time 2, time 2 to time 3 and time 1 to time 3 were available for 150, 127 and 130 cases respectively. As well as attrition due to deaths, missing cases resulted from a mixture of refusals, severe cognitive impairment and residents moving out of the homes before the end of the study. Of the 188 who were alive until time 3, 165 had a GDS score at time 1. The 23 GDS-12R scores missing at time 1 are accounted for by residents' severe cognitive impairment (n=20) and three other residents who refused to answer sufficient questions to calculate a score. There were 133 time 3 GDS-12R scores. The missing 32 scores from residents who had completed a time 1 GDS-12R score were because five residents had moved out, 12 refused to be interviewed at time 2 or 3, and 16 became too severely cognitive impaired. There was no significant difference between the GDS-12R scores at time 1 for those with and without a GDS-12R score at time 3, suggesting that there was no systematic difference in this respect between those who remained in the sample at time 3 and those who did not (t = -0.53, d.f. = 163, p = 0.595).

Figure 11.1 indicates that both negative and positive changes in depression scores occurred, but mean change scores of around zero mean that there was no systematic increase or decrease in depression over time for the survivors as a whole (Figure 11.2).

Sixty-three (38 per cent) were classified as depressed cases at time 1, using the GDS-12R. Of this group of 63 residents, the majority (75 per cent) were still depressed at time 2 and 61 per cent (n=32) at time 3. This level of continuing depression at nine months post admission is striking. According to the HONOS-65+ ratings made by staff, 50 per cent of residents identified by GDS-12R as depressed at time 3 were considered by staff to have no depression problem. Thus the picture for a significant number of residents was that they were depressed on admission, this was unrecognised by staff and they remained depressed nine months later.

In a detailed review of the literature on depression in care homes, Ames (1994) argued that since this is a largely treatable condition, there is no reason why rates of depression should not decrease after admission. He also highlighted the need to discriminate between three groups of residents — those whose depression is a key factor in the admission, those for whom depression is a response to admission and those who become depressed during their stay. In this study the first group could not be identified because pre-admission data were not collected. However assessment at admission and five months later identified the other two groups.

Figure 11.1
Changes in depression scores (GDS-12R) between time 1 and time 3

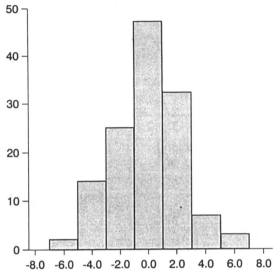

Figure 11.2
Changes in mean depression scores (GDS-12R)

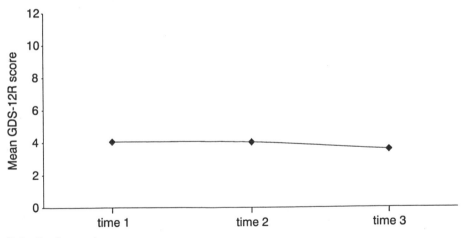

Note: Survivors only.

Of residents who were not depressed at time 1, 17 per cent (n=23) became depressed by time 2. Only 13 of these residents were assessed at time 3 for depression and only four of these remained depressed. Clearly, with such small numbers it is difficult to draw conclusions about the time 3 data. However, it is noteworthy that, of the 63 residents who were found to be depressed at time 2, 71 per cent had been depressed since admission compared with 29 per cent who became depressed after admission. This suggests that for those who were depressed on admission, either resulting from relocation or suffering from long-term depression, detection and/or treatment were not forthcoming within the homes.

Antidepressant medication was rarely prescribed to residents classed as depressed 'cases'. At time 1, only 19.1 per cent of depressed residents were prescribed antidepressants, although there appeared to be some increase over time (25.8 per cent at time 2 and 26.2 per cent at time 3). In about one-third of these cases antidepressant medication was being received in a dose below the usual therapeutic range. As Table 11.1 illustrates, at time 2, 15 per cent of those who were not depressed were being prescribed antidepressants — this may be evidence that the medication was working effectively, however one-fifth of these people were also receiving sub-therapeutic doses, some of which may have been maintenance doses. It would appear that, since the distribution is just less than would be expected by chance, the access to medication of residents requiring anti-depressants was low. In 89.7 per cent (n=35) of cases where both staff (using the HONOS-65+ ratings) and residents' responses (using GDS-12R) were indicative of depression, there was no antidepressant medication prescribed. This may suggest either that health care professionals take a fatalistic view of depression in older residents, regarding it as inevitable and untreatable and/or that there is poor communication between home staff and medical practitioners.

Heston et al. (1992) noted a similar tendency for older people in care homes with depression not to receive treatment. In their longitudinal study of

Table 11.1
Time 2 — depressed cases and receipt of medication

	No anti-depressants (%)	Antidepressant medication (%)	Dose	Total
Depressed cases	46	18	Includes	64
	(72%)	(28%)	therapeutic = 12 sub therapeutic = 6	
Non-depressed cases	78	14	Includes	92
	(85%)	(15%)	therapeutic = 11 sub therapeutic = 3	
Chi-Square = 3.857		p = 0.0495		

consecutive admissions to care homes, of a subgroup of 258 'alert and oriented' depressed residents identified on admission, two-thirds were still depressed one year later with only 13 per cent having received antidepressant medication, of whom 80 per cent had been given sub-therapeutic doses. Only 6 per cent of the treated group had medication initiated during their stay in the home.

This present study, therefore, supports other research findings that: levels of depression are high in nursing and residential homes; its recognition by staff is poor; and, perhaps most importantly, even when the presence of depression is recognised it often goes untreated.

Morale

Consistent with the pattern observed in the depression scores, there were few changes over time in the ten dimensions of the Affect Balance Scale (Table 11.2), with sizeable changes for only two dimensions. There was a decrease from 41 per cent to 21 per cent between times 1 and 2 in the percentage of residents responding 'yes' to the item asking about whether they were pleased that they had accomplished something.

Many of the residents — always more than 50 per cent — who completed this scale reported being bored at all three time periods. The lack of any improvement over time is noteworthy. At each interview those who reported being bored were significantly more depressed ($p \leq 0.0005$). Even when residents who had been depressed at time 1 were excluded from the analysis, residents who reported being bored at time 3 were significantly more depressed at that time ($p = 0.027$). Boredom or lack of interest is symptomatic of depression, and the reported boredom may be one manifestation of the underlying depressive disorder rather than a cause of it. However, this pattern is consistent with one observed in the multivariate analyses described below, and will be discussed further.

It is encouraging to note that the proportion of residents who felt lonely or remote from others decreased from 41 per cent at time 1 to around 27 per cent at time 3. This could suggest that following admission to the care homes, residents may have developed friendships or benefited from better contact with relatives and other visitors, or could indicate that those who survived to the third interview were more integrated with other residents, perhaps due to their lower dependency and frailty.

Dependency

There was no systematic increase in dependency scores for survivors as a whole (Figure 11.3). Mean Barthel scores were similar at all three assessment

Table 11.2
Responses to Affect Balance Scale Items at three time periods

Affect Balance Item		% yes (n)	% no (n)
Pleased that you've accomplished something	time 1	41.3 (n=43)	58.7 (n=61)
	time 2	21.2 (n=22)	78.8 (n=82)
	time 3	20.7 (n=18)	79.3 (n=69)
Things going your way	time 1	51.5 (n=52)	48.5 (n=49)
	time 2	52.5 (n=52)	47.5 (n=47)
	time 3	47.6 (n=39)	52.4 (n=43)
Been complimented	time 1	46.1 (n=47)	53.9 (n=55)
	time 2	34.7 (n=35)	65.3 (n=66)
	time 3	34.1 (n=29)	65.9 (n=56)
Excited or interested in something	time 1	26.9 (n=28)	73.1 (n=76)
	time 2	21.2 (n=22)	78.8 (n=82)
	time 3	20.7 (n=18)	79.3 (n=69)
On top of the world	time 1	22.9 (n=24)	77.1 (n=81)
	time 2	21.2 (n=22)	78.8 (n=82)
	time 3	22.2 (n=20)	77.8 (n=70)
Too restless to sit in a chair	time 1	38.7 (n=41)	61.3 (n=65)
	time 2	31.4 (n=33)	68.6 (n=72)
	time 3	30.0 (n=27)	70.0 (n=63)
Bored	time 1	59.4 (n=63)	40.6 (n=43)
	time 2	53.3 (n=56)	46.7 (n=49)
	time 3	54.9 (n=50)	45.1 (n=41)
Depressed or very unhappy	time 1	44.3 (n=47)	55.7 (n=59)
	time 2	41.9 (n=44)	58.1 (n=61)
	time 3	39.6 (n=36)	60.4 (n=55)
Lonely or remote from other people	time 1	41.1 (n=44)	58.9 (n=63)
	time 2	33.7 (n=35)	66.3 (n=69)
	time 3	27.5 (n=25)	72.5 (n=66)
Upset because criticised	time 1	10.4 (n=11)	89.6 (n=95)
	time 2	9.5 (n=10)	90.5 (n=95)
	time 3	7.9 (n=7)	92.1 (n=82)

Figure 11.3
Changes in dependency scores (Barthel)

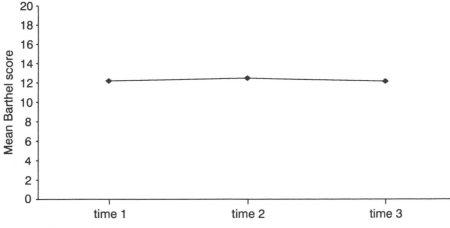

Note: Survivors only.

points (all around 12.5). None of the differences between scores at different points are close to the difference of 4 suggested by Collin et al. (1988) as indicative of clinically significant changes in levels of dependency.

Using the Barthel score groupings described in Chapter 5, Table 11.3 shows how the surviving residents moved between dependency groups over the nine months of the study. The majority were in the low dependency group on admission and remained there. Only 12 per cent of the low dependency survivors moved into a higher dependency group, indicating a high level of stability over the first nine months of care home residence.

In a significant number of residents there appears to have been some improvement during this period. Around one-third of the survivors moved from being classed as high or medium dependency to low or low / medium dependency. It seems unlikely that this was due simply to living in a specially

Table 11.3
Dependency groups at times 1, 2 and 3*

	Number (%) at time 1	Number (%) at time 2	Number (%) at time 3
High dependency	18 (11.4)	19 (12.0)	29 (18.4)
Medium dependency	30 (18.9)	20 (12.7)	17 (10.8)
Low/medium dependency	26 (16.5)	24 (15.2)	20 (12.7)
Low dependency	84 (53.2)	95 (60.1)	92 (58.2)

Note: * Based on residents with dependency information at each time point (n=158).

adapted environment. Although the residents were recently admitted, at the time of the first assessment, informant staff reported on residents' level of functioning in an environment with hand rails, lifts and other aids. It is more likely that this represents a genuine improvement, due to unknown factors that may well include beneficial aspects of the care being received as well as possible recuperative effects.

It may be recalled from Chapter 5 that a significant number of residents were classified as having low dependency needs on admission. Follow-up data indicate that there were no large group changes for the survivors. Of the 84 residents who were classed as 'low dependency' on admission 72 (86 per cent) remained so at the end of the study period.

Dependency group comparisons

Three groups of residents, who were distinct in terms of the stability of their dependency levels, were examined in greater detail. These were residents whose dependency scores improved during the nine months (n=20), residents who had consistently low levels of dependency throughout (n=68), and residents whose levels of dependency varied (n=75).

Source of admission Half (n=10) of the residents classed as 'improvers' had originally been admitted from hospital, eight of them to residential homes. Forty-four per cent of residents with varying dependency and 37 per cent of residents with consistently low dependency had also been admitted from hospital.

Cognitive ability Residents with higher time 1 scores on the MMSE (the less cognitively impaired), formed a higher proportion of the 'stable low dependency' and 'improvers' groups. Seventy-eight per cent (n=53) of residents in the stable low dependency group and 75 per cent (n=15) of residents classed as 'improvers' scored 10 or more. Residents of varying dependency were more equally spread on their original MMSE score, with 57.3 per cent scoring 10 or more (n=43).

Diagnosis Table 11.4 shows diagnoses according to dependency group. Several points are noteworthy:

Twenty-four per cent of those with varying levels of dependency had a diagnosis of dementia, compared with 10 per cent of the improvers and 16.2 per cent with stable low dependency. Doubts expressed earlier about the quality of this particular aspect of diagnostic information given to homes (Chapter 5) should, however, be recalled.

Table 11.4

Diagnoses for dependency groups

Diagnosis	% within changing dependency (n=75)	% within improvers (n=20)	% within stable dependency (n=68)
Cancer	none	5 (n=1)	2.9 (n=2)
Rheumatological	26.7 (n=20)	20 (n=4)	16.2 (n=11)
Dementia	24.0 (n=18)	10 (n=2)	16.2 (n=11)
Respiratory	6.7 (n=5)	10 (n=2)	10.3 (n=7)
Gastro-intestinal	5.3 (n=4)	5 (n=1)	10.3 (n=7)
Hepato-biliary	none	5 (n=1)	2.9 (n=2)
Kidney failure	none	none	none
Non-diabetic endocrine diagnosis	none	none	none
Diabetes	9.3 (n=7)	25 (n=5)	8.8 (n=6)
Neurological	20.0 (n=15)	none	8.8 (n=6)
Non-dementia psychiatric diagnosis	6.7 (n=5)	10 (n=2)	8.8 (n=6)
Dementia/neuro/other psychiatric diagnoses	44.0 (n=33)	20 (n=4)	32.4 (n=22)
Stroke	24.0 (n=18)	10 (n=2)	5.9 (n=4)
Stroke or rheumatological	49.3 (n=37)	25 (n=5)	22.1 (n=15)
Non-stroke cardiovascular	30.7 (n=23)	30 (n=6)	26.5 (n=18)
Cardiovascular (including stroke)	44.0 (n=33)	40 (n=8)	30.9 (n=21)

Twenty-four per cent of residents of variable dependency had suffered a stroke, compared with 10 per cent of improvers and 5.9 per cent of those with low, stable dependency scores.

Twenty-five per cent of the improvers had a diagnosis of diabetes, compared with 9.3 per cent of those with varying dependency and 8.8 per cent with stable and low dependency. The diagnostic information on this condition is believed to have been reasonably accurate. It seems possible that diabetics were heavily represented among the improvers because their diet and medication were better managed than before admission.

Cognitive impairment

There were minimal changes in MMSE scores over time for the survivors (Figure 11.4). For those who were severely impaired at time 1 (MMSE scores), the mean score change over the nine month period was 0.19, although it is worth noting that there was a wide range of change scores, from a decrease of 7 MMSE points to an increase of 12 points. For those with scores of 10 or over, the mean change in MMSE score was also low (–0.79). Once again, the range of

Figure 11.4
Changes in cognitive impairment over time (MMSE scores)

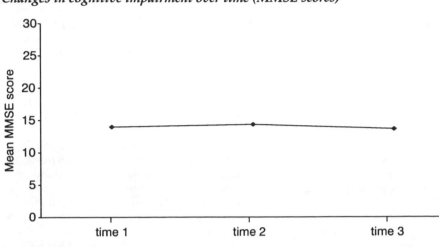

Note: Survivors only.

change scores was very wide, ranging from a decrease of 15 points to an increase of 9 points.

The fact that neither severely nor moderately cognitively impaired residents showed a high rate of decline over the study period supports the findings of Wild and Kaye (1998), who concluded that the rate of change in cognitive impairment was similar for both groups in their longitudinal study of cognitive impairment. Furthermore, they suggest that rates of subsequent decline in cognitive functioning cannot be related to baseline measures of impairment, at least over a period of nine months.

In this study there is evidence of change in survivors' MMSE scores for both those who entered the care homes with high levels and with low levels of cognitive impairment. However, these changes were in both directions and some of this may be due to measurement error. It is also possible that the MMSE scores on admission may have been affected by the admission process and it is notable that the change in MMSE scores from times 2 to 3 for the severely impaired group is considerably less varied. A similar picture emerges when specific domains of the MMSE are considered. Scores relating to residents' orientation to time and orientation to place (domains highlighted in Chapter 9) also move in both directions with mean change scores around zero.

As might be expected, the majority (80 per cent) of those who were assessed as severely cognitively impaired at time 1 continued to be so until time 3. An apparent anomaly is that eight residents classified at time 1 as severely cognitively impaired had markedly increased scores at both time 2 and time 3 — in three cases resulting in new scores of 16 or higher. Jacqmin-Gadda et al.

(1997) suggested that the testing situation itself might skew results. In their five-year longitudinal study they found that increased MMSE scores occurred in 'less educated' people (O'Connor et al., 1989), explaining the improvement as due to the stress of the test situation at time 1 and/or by a learning effect at time 2. It is also possible that residence in the home, perhaps by something as simple as improved and regular nutrition or reduced medication produced a genuine improvement in the cognitive functioning of these residents. Five of the eight had depression scores below the 'caseness' threshold of 5 (GDS-12R) at time 1 with the remaining three having scores of 5 (n=2) and 9. Thus depression at time 1 does not appear to account for the low initial MMSE scores.

Of the 128 surviving residents who were not assessed as severely cognitively impaired on admission, 18 (14 per cent) moved into this group by the end of the data collection period. Eighty-three per cent of this group had displayed moderate cognitive impairment (i.e. MMSE scores of less than 17) at time 1. Thus, the majority of residents who became severely cognitively impaired were already moderately impaired on admission.

Quality of life assessments

As Table 11.5 and Figures 11.5 to 11.10 illustrate (and as with the dependency and cognitive impairment measures), there was little variation over the nine-month follow-up period in any of the quality of life scales or sub-scales for survivors. Of these scales, at each time of administration the measures based on analogue scales (Cantril's ladder and the Spitzer Uniscale) were more widely distributed than the life satisfaction scores, indicating greater sensitivity, but variation over time was no greater. The lack of perceived change over time is less surprising than might be thought on initial observation. First, the data are only available for survivors, those people who adjusted to the admission to the homes and who had on average, lower levels of dependency and frailty. It might be hypothesised that changes in quality of life occur most markedly for those with the greatest health problems, who were least likely to survive. Second, the influence of home life upon residents' perceived quality of life is relatively homogeneous over time compared with the marked variability of factors influencing quality of life when they were in their own homes. Hence, apparent lack of variation in quality of life may be due to the greater similarity of experiences for residents in care homes, and to discriminate the key impact of a care home upon quality of life may require more minutely sensitive quality of life measures.

Table 11.5
Changes in quality of life measures

		Mean	s.d.	N
Life satisfaction score	time 1	4.00	0.448	110
	time 2	4.00	0.532	110
	time 3	3.95	0.549	91
Living situation satisfaction score	time 1	4.07	0.617	109
	time 2	4.06	0.599	110
	time 3	4.04	0.664	92
Life as a whole today	time 1	4.09	1.03	121
	time 2	4.01	1.04	113
	time 3	4.09	0.96	100
Life satisfaction as a whole	time 1	3.83	0.72	115
	time 2	3.83	0.82	113
	time 3	3.75	0.76	97
Leisure satisfaction	time 1	3.85	0.670	113
	time 2	3.93	0.728	108
	time 3	3.95	0.646	95
Health satisfaction	time 1	3.82	0.775	108
	time 2	3.86	0.809	106
	time 3	3.92	0.779	89
Satisfaction with living here a long time	time 1	4.20	4.180	187
	time 2	4.33	4.167	184
	time 3	4.45	4.181	167
Satisfaction with relative contact	time 1	4.25	0.79	106
	time 2	4.16	0.99	102
	time 3	4.07	0.98	94
Satisfaction with social contact	time 1	4.22	0.610	106
	time 2	4.20	0.679	106
	time 3	4.20	0.710	89
Satisfaction with religion	time 1	3.84	0.888	99
	time 2	3.90	0.821	98
	time 3	3.82	0.960	81
Satisfaction with money	time 1	3.65	0.986	93
	time 2	3.73	0.949	97
	time 3	3.89	1.092	79
Self concept score	time 1	0.73	0.227	99
	time 2	0.67	0.262	87
	time 3	0.65	0.219	72
Cantril's ladder	time 1	33.02	21.74	112
	time 2	31.60	23.39	104
	time 3	34.86	25.73	96
Spitzer Uniscale	time 1	39.73	17.11	188
	time 2	39.89	16.59	184
	time 3	39.64	17.91	166

Figure 11.5
Changes in Life Satisfaction score over time

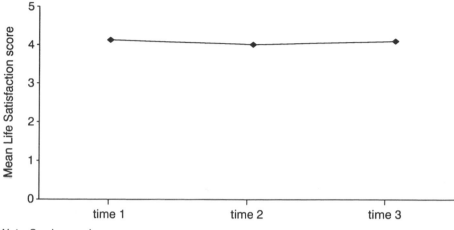

Note: Survivors only.

Figure 11.6
Changes in Leisure Satisfaction score over time

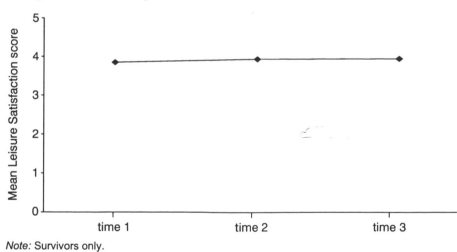

Note: Survivors only.

Figure 11.7
Changes in Health Satisfaction score over time

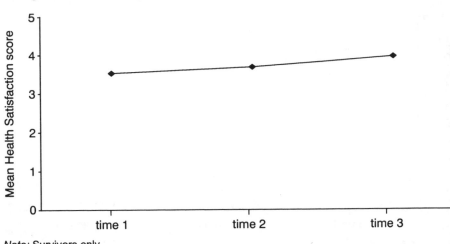

Note: Survivors only.

Figure 11.8
Changes in Satisfaction with Living Situation score over time

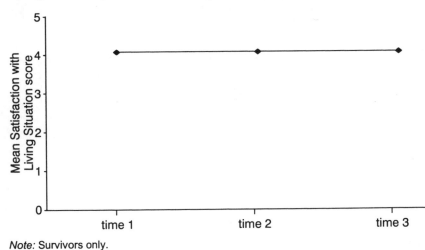

Note: Survivors only.

Figure 11.9
Changes in Spitzer Uniscale score over time

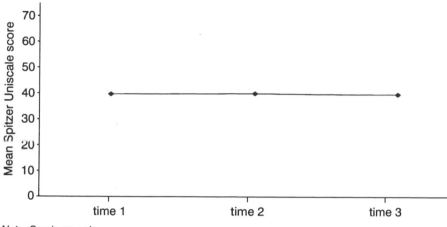

Note: Survivors only.

Figure 11.10
Changes in Cantril's ladder score over time

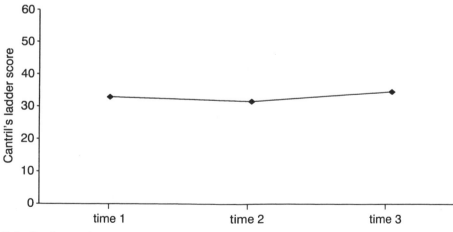

Note: Survivors only.

Changes in prescribed medication

Medication data were collected at all three assessments by consulting staff or home records. Compliance was almost universal — prescription of a medication in these care homes usually being equivalent to its actual receipt.

The mean number of prescribed drugs for newly admitted residents was 4.2 (std.dev. = 2.7, range 0–13). This figure did not fluctuate greatly across the three periods, with means and standard deviations of 4.6 and 2.9 respectively at both times 2 and 3. Only eight of the residents at time 1 received no drugs at all, and this figure remained virtually unchanged across all three time periods. At time 1, 40.5 per cent of residents were prescribed five or more drug items and this had increased to 46 per cent of residents by time 3.

These figures indicate lower levels of prescribing than previously reported in two studies, one from the north-west of England (Lunn et al., 1997) another from Northamptonshire (Corbett, 1997) where means of 7.1 and 6.5 prescribed items (range 0–15 and 0–14 respectively) were reported. The figures are, however, similar to those found in a medication review trial carried out in Manchester nursing homes, where numbers of drugs prescribed per resident were 5.1 and 4.9 for cases and controls respectively at baseline, and 4.4 and 4.2 respectively at final follow-up (Furniss et al., 2000).

There was no significant difference between nursing (mean 4.3) and residential homes (mean 3.9) in the number of drugs prescribed to residents, nor between residents admitted from the community or another home and those admitted from hospital. As in the study conducted by Primrose et al. (1987) there was no significant relationship between the age of the resident and the number of drugs taken.

The use of central nervous system drugs was notably high. At time 1, 68.9 per cent of residents were prescribed such drugs and this figure continued to rise — to 76 per cent and 78.3 per cent of residents at times 2 and 3 respectively. It should, however, be noted that analgesics such as paracetamol (but not aspirin) were included in this group.

Psychotropic medication was prescribed to 30.8 per cent of residents at time 1, 34.5 per cent at time 2 and 29.2 per cent at time 3. Figure 11.11 illustrates the changes in prescribing pattern by specific drug category and it can be seen that the prescription of night-time minor and major tranquillisers decreased with time, while the other psychotropic drugs increased, in at least one of the time periods.

At time 1, 35.5 per cent of residents were prescribed laxatives, a rate similar to that reported in Edinburgh by Primrose et al. (1987) but markedly different from more recent studies in the US where figures of laxative consumption by older people in nursing homes have been reported to have been as high as 74.6 per cent (Pahor et al., 1994). There was an increase in the percentage of residents prescribed laxatives by time 2, when 45.9 per cent (n=90) of residents

Figure 11.11
Changes in prescribed psychotropic medication over time

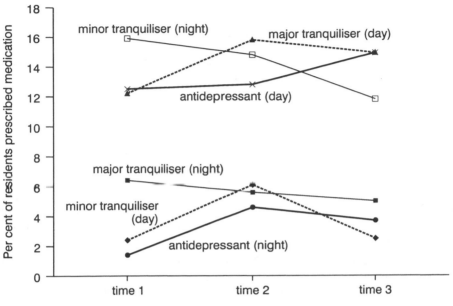

Note: Survivors only.

were prescribed such items, although this figure reduced slightly by time 3 (41 per cent, n=66). At time 3 nursing home residents were significantly (χ^2 $p < 0.001$) more likely to be prescribed laxatives than residential home residents, with rates of 57.5 per cent and 27.3 per cent respectively.

Relatives' satisfaction

As described in Chapter 8, there were two ratings of relatives' satisfaction. The first recorded satisfaction with the care given to the resident. The second referred to the home's cleanliness, appearance and comfort. Unfortunately, the response rates for these scales at times 2 and 3 were very low and the following data must be viewed with that in mind.

Sixty-six scores were available for the first satisfaction scale at times 1 and 2. Of these, 85 per cent were very happy when asked on admission of their relative, and 80 per cent of this group remained happy at time 2. No relatives reported that they were 'unhappy' with the care on either occasion. There were only 71 relatives who answered the question regarding satisfaction with the presentation and cleanliness of the home at both times 1 and 2. From this sample, 88.3 per cent were 'very satisfied' on both occasions. There were only two relatives who suggested that they were dissatisfied, and one who changed from being very satisfied to being 'neither satisfied nor dissatisfied'.

Factors influencing residents' survival

This issue is explored in two ways. Comparisons are first made between resident 'survival groups'; this is followed by a Cox proportional hazards regression analysis of factors predicting survival using augmented survival data collected about one year after the end of the study period.

The three 'survival groups'

These three groups were defined as follows:

* *Survival Group 1:* Those who were alive throughout the study — seen at all three data collection points: on admission (time 1), five months (time 2) and nine months post admission (time 3).
* *Survival Group 2:* Those residents who died between five and nine months post admission.
* *Survival Group 3:* Those residents who died between admission and the five-month follow up.

Survival data were available for 258 out of the 308 residents (84 per cent). The remaining 50 (16 per cent) residents either moved out of the home before the final stage of data collection (9 per cent) or refused further contact after the initial interview (7 per cent).

The majority of residents (72.9 per cent of known cases) survived throughout the nine month data collection period. As might be expected, given the generally higher degree of dependency in nursing homes (see Chapter 5), the majority of deaths (71.5 per cent) occurred here. Seventy-five per cent of deaths occurred within five months of admission. This is illustrated in Figure 11.12.

Table 11.6 provides data on survival groups in relation to a number of variables. There was no significant difference in age between the three survival groups nor was there an association between sex of the resident and death. However there was a difference between men and women in the timing of death with men more likely to die sooner. The mean survival time for women was 134 days compared to 76 days for men.

There was no significant difference in survival time for residents from the different admission sources. Although 47 per cent of those who died had been admitted to a care home from hospital (33 out of 70 non-survivors) this figure was not dissimilar to the proportion of survivors (43.6 per cent) admitted from

Figure 11.12
Hazard plot — survival of nursing and residential home residents

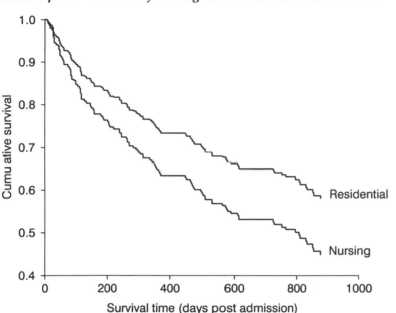

hospital (82 out of 188 survivors). It might have been expected that those going into nursing or residential homes directly from hospital would differ from the others, but no such difference was found.

It was difficult to acquire reliable information on causes of death. Although staff in participating homes were asked directly for this information, often they either did not know or gave incomplete responses. This does not indicate lack of co-operation by staff; rather that cause of death information in general is known to be problematic (Newens et al., 1993; Devis and Rooney, 1997). When death occurs in later life 'old age' may be seen as an acceptable cause to record. In a study of over 2000 nursing home deaths Robertson (1996) found that this could apply between the ages of 69 and 106 years! Even if good quality data for this study had been available, it would be difficult to make comparisons with national figures since death rate statistics are not available separately for nursing and residential homes for the elderly (Office of National Statistics, 2000). The category covering nursing and residential homes also includes 'maternity homes, holiday homes, homes for the disabled, hostels and other hospitals'. However, the death rate of 30 per cent (over nine months) found in this study is similar to that reported by Bebbington et al. (1996).

Table 11.6
Survival group — demographic data

Variable	Group 1 Survived	Group 2 Died between time 2 and time 3	Group 3 Died between time 1 and time 2	Refused or moved out	N (%)
Home Type					
Nursing	84 (53.2%)	12 (7.6%)	38 (24.1%)	24 (15.2%)	158 (100%)
Residential	104 (69.3%)	5 (3.3%)	15 (10.0%)	26 (17.3%)	150 (100%)
Sex					
Male	55 (57.3%)	2 (2.1%)	22 (22.9%)	17 (17.7%)	96 (100%)
Female	133 (62.7%)	15 (7.1%)	31 (14.6%)	33 (15.6%)	212 (100%)
Mean age at admission					
(years)	83.16	84.64	82.22	81.60	308
Admission source					
Own home	50 (53.8%)	2 (2.2%)	20 (21.5%)	21 (22.6%)	93 (100%)
Relatives home	12 (54.5%)	1 (4.5%)	3 (13.6%)	6 (27.3%)	22 (100%)
Hospital	82 (60.7%)	11 (8.1%)	22 (16.3%)	20 (14.8%)	135 (100%)
Residential home	28 (75.7%)	2 (5.4%)	5 (13.5%)	2 (5.4%)	37 (100%)
Nursing home	16 (76.2%)	1 (4.8%)	3 (14.3%)	1 (4.8%)	21 (100%)
Geographic areas					
Manchester	24 (55.8%)	1 (2.3%)	12 (27.9%)	6 (14.0%)	43 (100%)
Cheshire	95 (64.6%)	12 (8.2%)	18 (12.2%)	22 (15.0%)	147 (100%)
Blackpool	69 (58.5%)	4 (3.4%)	23 (19.5%)	22 (18.6%)	118 (100%)

'Survival group' physical health comparisons Differences in measures of physical well-being were found between the three survival groups, using the indicators of the Barthel and Crichton Royal scores, diagnoses and current prescribed medication.

The mean Barthel scores on admission for each survival group were 12.19 for the survivors (Group 1), 11.35 for those who died after time 2 (Group 2) and 8.52 for those who died after time 1 (Group 3). Only the difference between Groups 1 and 3 was statistically significant (p 0.001). A similar statistically significant difference was found between the same groups when using the Crichton Royal as a dependency measure (p = 0.005). This adds confidence to the conclusion that those who died soonest had the highest measured dependency on admission. The usefulness of the Barthel as an indicator of physical health will be further discussed in Chapter 12.

There was a bigger increase in dependency (Barthel) from time 1 to time 2 for those who died than for those who survived throughout and for those who died between time 2 and time 3. This difference was significant in spite of the fact that change scores were only available for 15 of the residents who died. The mean Barthel score change for the survivors was 0.46 compared with –2.0 for those who died (t = 2.8, p = 0.005). The negative value indicates that physical dependency increased overall for this group between time 1 and time 2. However, a change of 2 points on a scale ranging between 0 and 20 is not necessarily of clinical significance (Collin et al., 1988) and this must be viewed with caution.

The quality of the diagnosis data was found not to be consistent across the homes. Moreover the low levels of diagnosed illness in many categories made comparisons difficult. In terms of the drug categories used in this study (Chapter 5) there were no striking differences between the survival groups.

'Survival group' mental health comparisons There was no significant difference in time 1 MMSE score between survivors and those who died. In terms of the *change* in MMSE scores, there was, however, a significant difference between the few residents who died between times 2 and 3 and the survivors. There was virtually no change in the surviving group, compared with a reduction in score of nearly 3 points (on a 30 point scale) in those who died between times 2 and 3 (t = 2.94, d.f. 181, p = 0.003). Again this is a relatively small change but given the short period of time both the direction of change and the significance level is worth noting. Decline in cognitive functioning was thus associated with non-survival.

Residents who died before the five-month follow-up were more depressed than those who survived longer. The time 1 GDS-12R mean score for this group was 5.33 compared with 2.64 for those who died between five and nine months and 4.06 for nine month survivors — differences which were statistically significant (F = 4.805, p = 0.009).

'Survival group' quality of life comparisons When the three 'survival' groups were compared individually with the quality of life ratings, there were significant differences between the groups for Life Satisfaction Scale total score, and Health Satisfaction Sub-scale. These are shown in Table 11.7. Interestingly the differences between the groups were greatest between those who died soonest, having the lowest mean satisfaction scores for both variables, and those who died between time 2 and 3 having the highest mean satisfaction scores. The survivor group had mean satisfaction scores which came somewhere in between for both variables. Investigation of the explanation for this is beyond the scope of the present study. However, a considerable literature has examined the impact of entry to care homes on frail older people. Differential impact of the move on these individuals is often

Table 11.7
Survival group and quality of life variables

	Survivors	Died between time 1 and time 2	Died between time 2 and time 3	F	p
LSS	3.97 (n=110)	3.64 (n=32)	4.31 (n=11)	9.34	<0.001
Cantril's ladder	33.02 (n=112)	36.50 (n=24)	19.55 (n=11)	2.43	ns
Health Satisfaction sub-scale	3.82 (n=108)	3.35 (n=31)	4.10 (n=10)	5.19	0.007
Spitzer Uniscale	39.73 (n=188)	32.15 (n=53)	37.18 (n=17)	3.99	0.02

	Survivors	Died before time 3		F	p
LSS	3.97 (n=110)	3.81 (n=43)		3.00	ns
Cantril's ladder	33.02 (n=112)	31.17 (n=35)		0.19	ns
Health Satisfaction sub-scale	3.82 (n=108)	3.54 (n=41)		3.61	ns
Spitzer Uniscale	39.73 (n=188)	33.37 (n=70)		6.90	0.009

Note: Cantril's ladder: low score = good life.

associated with their own health status, the degree of preparation for the move and the degree to which they perceive entry to the home as predictable and within their control (Lieberman, 1961; Yawney and Slover, 1973; Tobin and Lieberman, 1976; Schultz and Brenner, 1977). The Spitzer Uniscale also showed a significant difference between the three survival groups, however in this case interviewer ratings indicated that those who died soonest had the lowest mean quality of life scores, and survivors had the highest mean quality of life scores.

There were no significant differences in any of the main self-reported quality of life ratings — Life Satisfaction Scale total score, Cantril's ladder or the Health Satisfaction Sub-scale between those who survived throughout (Survival Group 1) and those who died at any time before time 3 (Survival Groups 2 and 3). The Spitzer Uniscale (interviewer rated) did, however, show a significant difference between survivors and those who subsequently died

Predictors of survival — the survival analysis

Because most of the study residents remained alive throughout the nine-month follow-up period, changes could be analysed for a fairly large survivor group over nine months. However the mean survival time for older people in care homes has been estimated at around 12.3 months for nursing homes and 24 months for residential homes (Bebbington et al., 1996). Because nine months was, therefore, a relatively short time for studying predictors of survival, a telephone follow-up was carried out approximately one year after the end of the study and this survival analysis is based on this augmented data. It should be noted that the analysis was performed using the baseline data only. A number of those who died did so prior to the second wave of interviewing at time 2, but the time 1 data are available for the whole cohort.

Variables separately entered into the survival analysis included individual resident characteristics and environmental measures, all drawn from the list in Appendix 4. For those factors which were significant when entered singly, hazard ratios and significance levels are given in Table 11.8. The Health Satisfaction Sub-scale was made up of three satisfaction questions: How satisfied are you with — the state of your health?; how often you see a doctor?; the state of your nerves? That the Health Satisfaction Sub-scale score appears in this table is an interesting finding. It suggests that a simple self-rated assessment of health status or satisfaction may be as useful as more complex (and costly) ones. Earlier studies have noted a relationship between self-rated health, physician ratings, functional impairment and level of care (Johnson, 1972; Maddox and Douglas, 1973; Kraus et al., 1976). Interestingly, Maddox and Douglas (1973) found that self-rated health was a better predictor of future physical state than the physician rating.

Table 11.8
Factors associated with death when variables entered singly

	Model coefficient β	S.E.	d.f.	p value	Hazard ratio (exp β)	95% Confidence Interval for exp β
Barthel score	-0.0713	0.0164	1	< 0.0005	0.9312	0.9017 – 0.9616
MMSE score	-0.0268	0.0128	1	0.0366	0.9736	0.9495 – 0.9983
Spitzer Uniscale	-0.0197	0.0053	1	0.0002	0.9805	0.9704 – 0.9907
Health Satisfaction Sub-scale	-0.2838	0.1281	1	0.0268	0.7529	0.5858 – 0.9679
Diagnosis of cardiovascular disease (inc. stroke)	0.3901	0.1844	1	0.0344	1.4771	1.0291 – 2.1201
Diagnosis of cancer	1.1398	0.5098	1	0.0254	3.1260	1.1508 – 8.4910
Medication for infection	1.1759	0.3203	1	0.0002	3.2410	1.7301 – 6.0713
Medication for endocrine disorder	0.5862	0.2374	1	0.0136	1.7971	1.1284 – 2.8621

Table 11.9
Cox survival model indicating factors associated with death

	Model coefficient β	S.E.	d.f.	p value	Hazard ratio (exp β)	95% Confidence Interval for exp β
Barthel score (continuous score 0–20)	-0.070	0.017	1	p < 0.0005	0.932	0.901 – 0.965
Diagnosis of cancer	1.139	0.396	1	p = 0.0040	3.142	1.439 – 6.784
Prescribed medication for infections	1.148	0.321	1	p = 0.0004	3.151	1.679 – 5.913
Prescribed medication for the endocrine system	0.467	0.239	1	p = 0.0506	1.5958	0.999 – 2.547

Note: Chi-square =43.67 (4 d.f.) p < 0.0001

Because the Barthel was the most highly significant of these predictors of death, in the next stage of analysis this variable was combined with the others. The collinearity of the Barthel with many of the other variables reduced the number of variables that contributed to survival in this analysis. Table 11.9 shows the variables included in this final model, with hazard ratios and significance levels. These were dependency (with higher Barthel scores/lower dependency increasing survival likelihood), diagnosis of cancer (diagnosis decreasing survival likelihood), prescription of drugs to treat infection, and prescription of endocrine system drugs (receipt of these drugs linked with lower survival likelihood). Prescription of drugs was used as a proxy indicator of the presence of diseases because the diagnosis data was considered to be much more unreliable than the medication records. Separation of the endocrine system drugs into specific conditions such as diabetes, thyroid related conditions and those requiring steroids did not produce significant associations. However, this is likely to be due to the small numbers of cases resulting from such division. It is important to note that these four variables — dependency, cancer diagnosis, infection drugs and endocrine drugs — each made an independent contribution to predicting survival.

Although home type (nursing or residential) appeared to be closely associated with survival, this was explained by the different levels of dependency within each type. In a study of long-term care residents, Flacker and Kiely (1998) also found that their measure of functional impairment was the key survival predictor. They usefully warn that this association is not necessarily causal; rather that such a variable is useful to identify populations at risk. Thus dependency is probably best regarded as a manifestation of underlying problems that reduce survival, rather than as causative in itself. However, while taking steps to reduce dependency might not, in itself, have an effect in increasing survival, identifying dependency properly might allow professionals to target care more appropriately.

Survival of residents able to do quality of life interview at time 1 (MMSE>9) A separate survival analysis was performed for those residents who completed a quality of life interview. Since the criterion for this was an MMSE score of 10 or higher the following applies only to those without severe cognitive impairment.

As well as the Barthel score two further variables were identified as contributing to survival for this group. These were satisfaction with leisure in the home and receipt of drugs for cardiovascular disease (receipt of such drugs reducing the likelihood of survival). The variable relating to satisfaction with leisure in the home was examined further and the single item 'how satisfied are you with the pleasure you get from things you do here in the home?' was found to have most predictive value. The relationship, although small, indicated that increased likelihood of survival was associated with a higher level of

Table 11.10

Cox survival model — factors associated with death for those with MMSE scores >9 (i.e. excluding the most severely cognitively impaired) in the first nine months

	Model coefficient β	S.E.	d.f.	p value	Hazard ratio (exp β)	95% Confidence Interval for exp β
Barthel score (continuous score 0–20)	-0.091	0.026	1	p = 0.0003	0.9139	0.869 – 0.960
Level of pleasure experienced in the home	-0.405	0.117	1	p = 0.0005	0.667	0.531 – 0.839
Cardiovascular system	0.686	0.0323	1	p = 0.0338	1.9849	1.054 – 3.739

Note: Chi-square = 26.79 (3 d.f.), p < 0.0001.

expressed pleasure. This variable had a significant effect both singly (p = 0.0012) and in the presence of the Barthel score (p = 0.0005) (Table 11.10).

It is interesting to note that in this study depression (as assessed by the GDS-12R) was not linked to survival. This contrasts with several reported studies (for example, Murphy et al., 1988) in which, even when physical illness was controlled for, depressed older people were more likely to die. There were also notable differences between these findings and those of Bebbington et al. (1998), who found that sex, age, depression, source of admission and respiratory illness were all factors affecting survival.

Care environment influences on outcome

To analyse the extent to which aspects of the care environment had an impact on residents' mental and physical functioning and quality of life, home level variables were related to individual level variables representing resident outcomes. In some cases individual level variables other than the one being used as the outcome were also included as predictors, for example in checking whether in predicting depression at time 3 any environmental factors remained significant, or were overridden when controlling for physical dependency. All these individual and home level variables were again drawn from the list provided in Appendix 4.

Outcome 1: physical functioning at nine months (time 3)

Physical functioning outcome measure — Barthel dependency score As reported above, there was no significant change in the Barthel scores of survivors over the nine-month period of the study. Regression analysis using the time 3 Barthel score as the dependent variable produced no significant relationships with any of the home level variables used to represent aspects of the care environment. The study does not, therefore, indicate that there are aspects of care that have a particular impact on dependency one way or the other, at least viewed over a period of nine months. It is, however, possible that residence in a home — any of the homes — had such an impact. There was no evidence of general reduction in dependency during the period of care to provide any indication that homes have rehabilitative effects. However there was no general increase in dependency either, and it could be argued that, for residents receiving long-term care, maintenance of the status quo — prevention of deterioration — is a real success.

Physical functioning outcome measure — health satisfaction score This health rating made by the residents themselves was examined as an additional indication of physical functioning, but was only available for residents who scored 10 or more on the MMSE, because it formed part of the quality of life interview. Linear regression using the time 3 health satisfaction score as the dependent variable revealed three variables as significant predictors, namely the depression (GDS-12R) score at time 3, the Sheltered Care Environment Scale *physical comfort* sub-scale and the Spitzer Uniscale. Thus the only care environment measure which contributed to this evaluation of health was the physical comfort of the surroundings as judged by staff. The major predictor of low satisfaction with health was being depressed, but even when this was controlled for, the home's physical comfort remained significant (Table 11.11). Other 'resident level' indicators of physical well-being were not associated with health satisfaction at time 3. These included the Barthel, diagnosis of disease or prescription of disease specific drugs (used as proxy indicators of disease).

Table 11.11
Factors relating to health perceptions at time 3 (nine months post admission) for those with MMSE scores >9 (i.e. excluding the most severely cognitively impaired)

	Model coefficient	S.E.	t	p value
Depression at time 3	-0.116	0.025	-4.598	0.008
SCES Comfort score	0.017	0.008	20.82	0.041
Spitzer Uniscale	0.023	0.006	3.849	≤ 0.0005
Constant	1.99	0.74	2.700	0.008

F=23.49   p<0.0001
$R^2 = 0.47$ Adjusted $R^2 = 0.45$

Outcome 2: mental functioning at nine months (time 3)

Mental functioning outcome measure — depression (GDS-12R score) It should be recalled here that depression scores were not available for the most severely cognitively impaired residents (Chapter 5). Linear regression using the time 3 GDS-12R score as the dependent variable produced four variables which were significant in predicting depression at time 3 (Table 11.12). These were:

- depression at time 1 (being depressed at time 1 predicted being depressed at time 3);
- dependency at time 3 (high concurrent dependency measured by the Barthel predicted depression at time 3);
- satisfaction at time 2 with the 'pleasure you get from things you do here in the home' (low satisfaction at time 2 predicted depression at time 3);

Table 11.12

Factors relating to depression at time 3 (nine months post admission) for those with MMSE scores >9 (i.e. excluding the most severely cognitively impaired)

	Model coefficient	S.E.	t	p value
Dependency (Barthel) at time 3	-0.113	0.041	-2.736	0.008
Depression at time 1	0.531	0.067	7.983	≤ 0.0005
Pleasure in the home at time 2	-1.514	0.510	-2.968	0.004
Opportunities to occupy self at time 2	-1.080	0.448	-2.409	0.018
Constant	5.146	0.824	6.24	<0.001

F= 35.62   p < 0.0001
R^2 = 0.64   Adjusted R^2 = 0.63

- satisfaction at time 2 with the 'opportunities for keeping yourself occupied here in the home' (low satisfaction at time 2 predicted depression at time 3).

Thus even when controlling both for depression on admission and for the current level of physical functioning, pleasure in the home and satisfaction with opportunities to occupy oneself were related to depression at time 3. It will be recalled that the 'pleasure in the home' variable featured as a predictor of survival and it is noteworthy that it appears again here.

Mental functioning outcome measure — cognitive impairment (MMSE score) None of the variables used to represent aspects of the care environment was significant in predicting cognitive impairment at time 3.

Outcome 3: Quality of life at nine months (time 3)

Quality of life outcome measures — Living situation satisfaction score; Cantril's ladder; Spitzer Uniscale When linear regression techniques were used to examine the care environment variables in relation to each of these quality of life measures in turn, there were no environmental factors that were significant as predictors of outcome.

Quality of life outcome measure — Satisfaction with the prospect of living here for a long time The only quality of life indicator which showed a relationship with environmental factors was the answer (given on a five-point scale) to this single question. This question produced more variability of response than any of the other 'living situation sub-scale' items; indeed more than any of the other items on the whole LQOLP-R interview (see Chapter 5 and Table 5.4).

Logistic regression using the time 3 response to this question as the dependent variable produced two significant predictors, one of which was a care environment measure:

• whether or not the home was in the 'positive' cluster (residents in 'positive' cluster homes being more likely to be satisfied with the prospect of remaining there);
• depression (GDS-12R) at time 3 (residents with lower levels of depression being more likely to be satisfied with the prospect of remaining there).

Together these two variables correctly predicted 79 per cent of responses to this question.

The clusters referred to were created using the procedure outlined in Chapter 7 and based on the Sheltered Care Environment Scale, which had been completed by staff in the homes. Positive cluster homes were those which had low scores for the *conflict* sub-scale and high scores for *cohesion*. The other characteristics of these clusters are discussed in Chapter 7 and illustrated in Table 7.4. Cluster 3 contained the *positive*, or perceived high quality homes. For purposes of the logistic regression described here, Clusters 1 and 2 were treated as one group so that the environmental variable becomes a binary one — membership or otherwise of the *positive* Cluster 3. As Table 11.13 indicates, being resident in such a home greatly increases the chances of being satisfied with the prospect of staying there for a long period of time. The Sheltered Care Environment Scale, completed by staff, embodies a staff view of what life is like for residents in the home. The *positive* cluster, it may be recalled from Chapter 7, correlated with the researchers' judgement of high quality — not perfectly, but reasonably well. It appears, therefore, that the logistic regression identifies a degree of congruence between the views of staff, researchers and residents about what constitutes a good home.

In summary

• Survival data were available for 258 of 308 residents. The majority of residents survived (72.9 per cent) throughout the nine-month period. The majority of deaths (71.5 per cent) occurred in nursing homes, and 75 per cent occurred in the first five months.
• The mean number of prescribed drugs for newly-admitted residents was 4.2 and this varied little over time. There were no significant differences between nursing and residential homes in the number of drugs prescribed. Around one-third of residents were prescribed psychotropic drugs at each time period.

Table 11.13

Factors relating to satisfaction with prospect of living in the home for a long time (nine months post admission) for those with MMSE scores >9 (i.e. excluding the most severely cognitively impaired)

	Model coefficient β	S.E.	Wald	p value	Hazard ratio (exp β)	95% Confidence Interval for exp β
Depression at time 3	-0.3506	0.0950	13.62	0.0002	0.7042	0.585–0.848
Home classified in the 'positive' cluster	1.4431	0.5234	7.60	0.0058	4.2337	1.5178–11.810
Constant	1.3981	0.5275	7.02	0.08		

Goodness of fit = 85.70
% correct prediction = 79.1%

- There were few changes over time on the 10-item Affect Balance Scale. However, over 50 per cent of residents who completed the scale reported being bored at each time period. At each interview those who reported being bored were also significantly more depressed.
- Anti-depressant medication was rarely prescribed to residents identified as depressed. In almost 90 per cent of cases where residents were judged by both themselves and staff to be depressed, no antidepressant medication was prescribed.
- Overall there was no systematic increase or decrease in depression over time for survivors. However, of 63 residents classed as depressed (GDS-12R) at time 1, 75 per cent were still depressed at time 2, and 61 per cent at time 3. Of those classed as depressed at time 3, half of them were rated by staff (HONOS-65+) as having no problems with depression.
- Four variables predicted depression at nine months; depression at time 1; dependency at time 3; lack of satisfaction with 'pleasure from things you do in the home' at time 2, and dissatisfaction at time 2 with 'opportunities for keeping yourself occupied'.
- There was no increase in dependency scores for survivors as a whole, using the Barthel. There were minimal changes in MMSE scores over time and little variation over time in any of the quality of life scales or sub-scales.
- Mean Barthel scores on admission for each survival group showed that those who died sooner had the highest dependency on admission. Analysis of variables independently associated with survival showed that higher dependency (using Barthel score), diagnosis of cancer, prescription of endocrine system drugs and drugs to treat infection, decreased likelihood of survival.
- Survival analysis on those residents who completed a quality of life interview showed that a higher level of dependency indicated by Barthel score, less satisfaction with leisure in the home, and receipt of cardiovascular disease drugs contributed to a reduced likelihood of survival.
- The single quality of life indicator showing a relationship with environmental factors was 'satisfaction with the prospect of living here for a long time'. Satisfaction was associated with being in a *positive* home and with the absence of depression. Together these variables predicted 79 per cent of responses to this question.

12 Towards Quality Care in Care Homes

The Quality of Life Study was an ambitious and complex project. Its primary aim was, if not to answer, at least to throw significant light on a question that has engaged researchers in this field over a number of years — what makes a good care home for older people? It is time to draw together the various threads of this work and examine the extent to which it has helped to answer that question. The data collected also provided a body of information about the characteristics of people now being admitted to care homes and about the staff who care for them, as well as giving rise to a number of subsidiary analyses. Drawing on all these data, some of the study's implications for social and health care policy are highlighted in this chapter.

Measuring outcomes for residents — some lessons learned

During the course of this study a number of measurement issues were encountered which may inform future work in this area. The first of these was the importance of inclusivity when selecting participants to interview about their situation. Many research studies exclude people with significant cognitive impairment and rely on proxies to act as informants. The work described in Chapter 9 demonstrates that many residents who would, in many research projects, be excluded from direct interviewing, were in fact able to give their own views about the services they received. This experience makes a strong case for being as inclusive as possible, and for great caution in using either carer opinions or global assessment scores such as the MMSE to make decisions about whether or not someone is able to be interviewed. This is particularly relevant with regard to the perspective of service users in service development and evaluation. Important examples include the acquisition of consumer satisfaction information (Cm 4169, 1998) and the place of the user perspective in the Single Assessment Process (SAP) in relation to the issue of capacity in decision-making (Department of Health, 2002a).

A second issue was the need to tailor scales or question items to the target population. An example of this is the development of the GDS-12R (Sutcliffe et al., 2000) to assess depression in residents of care homes, reported in Chapter 10. The new, adapted scale appeared to be a more effective assessment tool for the people interviewed in this study. By dropping some context-specific items, the scale became more sensitive to measurement and more acceptable to respondents.

Third, the study suggests that, at least when used in this context, global measures of quality of life may be relatively insensitive to change. Compared to domain-specific measures for instance, some of the individual domain questions were powerful outcome predictors in their own right. For example, satisfaction with pleasure from leisure activities and with the opportunities to keep occupied were predictive of depression; satisfaction with the prospect of living in the home for a long time was related to being in a *positive* home. As single items these are easier to administer than scales and should, perhaps, be included in future evaluative work where users' views are sought, or in a wider domain, for example in surveys of quality and user satisfaction (Cm 4169, 1998).

Fourth, as mentioned in Chapter 5, the interviewers noted some of the reluctance to express dissatisfaction which has been reported in other research with older people (Cartwright, 1964; Locker and Dunt, 1978; Wilkin and Hughes, 1987; Redfern, 1990; Geron, 1998). However, when responses to individual satisfaction questions were dichotomised, so as to group the neutral mid-point 'mixed/uncertain' with 'mostly' or 'very' dissatisfied, this reflected the way in which the scoring system appeared to be used by respondents. If these questions had been asked in 'yes/no' form it seems likely that very little dissatisfaction would have been expressed. The two stage process used here, in which respondents were asked to respond to a 'Likert' scale, with these responses subsequently collapsed into two categories, appeared to give a more accurate picture of their real feelings.

Lastly, mental health is an important consideration in the quality of life of older people. The relatively common problems of dementia and depression must be taken into account in any assessment of quality of life. It has been suggested (Challis, 1981) that depression, or more specifically its absence, can be seen as a proxy measure of quality of life, or at least of one of its component parts, namely subjective well-being. This approach was found to be of value in this study.

Factors contributing to a good outcome for residents

The search for possible contributions to outcome made by aspects of the care environment required separate investigation of survivors and non-survivors. Since death itself is an outcome it was important to detect any such factors which might predict non-survival as well as factors that predicted outcome in terms of mental and physical functioning and quality of life for those who survived throughout the study period.

In Chapter 1 four criteria were identified as almost self-evident components of a good outcome of care. These were physical functioning, mental health, cognitive functioning and quality of life. In addition the present study has identified the importance of relatives and home staff. In this chapter the evidence relating to each of these factors is summarised.

Survival

The most significant predictor of early death had nothing to do with the care environment. It was the individual's level of dependency on admission, whether measured by the Barthel or the Crichton Royal. Those who died soonest had the highest measured dependency on admission. The other variables — having a cancer diagnosis or receipt of drugs to treat infection or endocrine disorders — that were significantly associated with earlier death were also characteristics of the individual rather than of the home.

These findings are similar to those of a large scale retrospective study conducted over ten years with residents of an American nursing home (Breuer et al., 1998). Significant independent predictors of decreased survival included increased dependencies in activities of daily living and impairment of cardiac, respiratory, neurological and endocrine/metabolic systems. Cohen-Mansfield et al. (1999) found differences between cognitively intact and cognitively impaired residents. Significant predictors of survival in the former included more medical complaints and non-aggressive agitated behaviours, and in the latter, impaired activities of daily living and problem behaviours. As in the present study, depressed mood did not predict reduced survival in the Cohen-Mansfield study or in similar research carried out in residential homes in the Netherlands (Cuipers, 2001).

The only care environment factor related to survival was the response to the question 'how satisfied are you with the amount of pleasure you get from things you do here in the home?' and it is arguable that this too should be treated as an individual rather than an environmental characteristic. It suggests that where care home residents experience little pleasure in their daily life the outlook for them is poor. They are more likely to die early and more likely to be depressed. Although this question, included in the quality of life interview, was answered only by residents who scored 10 or more on the

MMSE, it is noteworthy that for these residents without severe cognitive impairment, deriving more pleasure from activities in the home was associated with greater likelihood of survival. This was the case even when Barthel measured dependency was taken into account.

When the nine-month outcomes were examined, for residents who remained alive throughout, there were no environmental variables which were significant predictors of cognitive impairment or dependency measured by the Barthel. The home *physical comfort* rating made by staff (Sheltered Care Environment Scale sub-scale) was a significant predictor of self-reported health satisfaction.

Physical functioning

It has been argued earlier in this book that good health, or even an individual's perception of good health, probably contributes more to overall quality of life than anything else (Denham, 1991). This present study supports the view that good physical health is related to good mental health and other positive outcomes. In this study, poorer physical health as defined by measures of dependency was associated with higher levels of depression, and those with higher levels of dependency survived for a shorter time.

It was apparent that individuals admitted to nursing homes with lower levels of dependency were more likely to be self-funding. This is consistent with a broader national study of self-funded residents which identified lower levels of dependency and cognitive impairment compared with publicly funded residents (Netten et al., 2002c). The majority of residents who survived throughout the study period were less dependent on admission and remained fairly stable over the nine months. Indeed a significant number of these residents became less dependent over time, which could suggest a genuine improvement in their health.

In this present study, seven out of ten residential home admissions and three out of ten nursing home admissions were individuals with low dependency needs. This raises a question about the targeting of scarce care home resources on those with the greatest needs, an important issue when personal resources become exhausted and public authorities need to decide upon the eligibility of a resident for a particular home. Factors in addition to those measured by the Barthel and Crichton Royal are important in assessing whether an individual requires admission to long-term care. This highlights the need for comprehensive assessment for older people prior to admission to long-term care (Challis et al., forthcoming) and for these services to be used for self-funding residents as well as those admitted with state support. Full implementation of the SAP could improve this situation (Department of Health, 2002a).

The high rate of prescription medication and polypharmacy in this study were similar to the findings in a number of other studies of nursing and residential homes conducted in the US (Gurvich and Cunningham, 2000; Sloane et al., 2002), and perhaps indicate a need for care home residents to have better access to expert and regular medication reviews, perhaps initiated by community pharmacists (Furniss et al., 2000). There is evidence that access for care home residents to both primary and secondary care services, including specialist mental health services, needs improvement (Jacobs et al., 2001; Challis et al., 2002b; Glendinning et al., 2002; Jacobs and Rummery, 2002).

Those who died soonest had the highest dependency on admission and those who died before the end of the nine-month study period showed an increase in dependency as measured by the Barthel. In light of the association between dependency and survival, identifying those residents with high dependency levels on admission may allow the targeting of appropriate care, and facilitate access to important external services.

Overall, there was no particular aspect of the care environment which had an impact on physical functioning over the nine months, and there was no evidence in the sample of residents as a whole of systematic changes in levels of dependency. Although there was no indication that the care homes had a rehabilitative effect on the residents, the lack of significant deterioration in their dependency levels could also be seen as a positive outcome in maintaining their physical functioning. It is possible that the study homes would have achieved a positive rehabilitative effect if they had used systematic exercise or fitness programmes such as those studied by Lazowski et al. (1999) and Richardson et al. (2001) or programmes to improve knowledge or awareness of care home staff (Gallichon, 2002).

Mental health

The presence of depressed mood or loneliness in substantial numbers of residents was similar to the findings of an American quality of life study (Ball et al., 2000). Just under half the residents in the present study expressed feelings of depression and loneliness, compared to more than half in the American study. In addition to the finding of high levels of depression generally, there was a significant association in the present study between depression and reduced mobility. For some residents, it was apparent that there was a high prevalence of co-morbidity of cognitive impairment and depression but no evidence of any such diagnosis. This highlights the need for care home residents to have access to specialist expertise in the diagnosis, treatment or management of these conditions (Audit Commission, 2000a; Jacobs et al., 2001; Challis et al., 2002b).

Generally, there were very low rates of recognition of depression around the time of admission by care staff, and there were no apparent differences between qualified nursing staff and unqualified staff in their rates of recognition. It was clear that even some residents with severe cognitive impairment were able to complete the depression measure with apparent validity. Of residents judged to be depressed on admission, most were still depressed at five months (time 2), and over 60 per cent at nine months (time 3). Of residents who remained depressed throughout the nine-month study period, only half were identified as depressed by staff. Thus a small but significant number of residents continued to be depressed, were unrecognised as such and remained untreated. A possible method of improving this situation is offered by Moxon et al. (2001) who have reported some success in training care staff in residential homes to identify depression and provide a care planning intervention for its management.

In the present study at admission, less than one in five residents found to be depressed (19 per cent) were receiving antidepressants. This situation had improved only slightly by five months (time 2) and nine months (time 3) where just over one quarter (26 per cent) of those classed as depressed were receiving antidepressants. These figures are even lower than those found in an Australian nursing home study where just 30 per cent of residents with significant depressive symptoms were prescribed antidepressants (Draper et al., 2001). More importantly, in almost 90 per cent of cases where there was agreement between staff and residents as to the presence of depression, no antidepressant medication was received. Although medication is not the only treatment for depression, it is possible that this indicates a poor level of communication between the care homes and primary care providers as well as lack of access to specialist services (cf. Department of Health, 2001b).

It appeared that those who died the soonest had been more depressed than those who survived for longer. Depression at time 3 (at the nine-month interview) was associated with depression at time 1 (admission), with concurrent high levels of dependency at time 3 and also with low levels of satisfaction with pleasure residents got from things they did in the home (at time 2). An important finding of the study was this link between certain aspects of the care environment and depression. For residents without severe cognitive impairment (MMSE 10+) depression at nine months post-admission was related to low satisfaction with 'the pleasure you get from things you do here in the home' and 'the opportunities for keeping yourself occupied here in the home'. These satisfaction levels were measured five months after admission, when residents had been able to recover from the immediate shock of relocation and form a considered view of the opportunities for occupation and pleasurable activity available to them in the homes. Even when the factors of high dependency and depression on admission were taken into account, low satisfaction in this area was a significant predictor of the poor outcome of being depressed. It may be worth recalling at this point the similar finding, reported in Chapter 11, that even when residents who had been depressed at time 1 were excluded, those who reported being bored at time 3 were significantly more depressed than those who did not. An American study of resident quality of life (Mitchell and Kemp, 2000) has also found an association between the care environment and depression. Although levels of depression were found to be far lower than in this present study, depression was found to be predicted by lack of social activities and by lower SCES *cohesion* scores (i.e. homes with staff who are less supportive and involved and residents who are less supportive of each other).

Cognitive functioning

Evidence from the Home Preliminary Questionnaire, completed by each of the home managers, indicated that the proportion of residents with cognitive impairment was higher in the study sample than in the total population of home residents. This suggests that those being admitted more recently were, on the whole, more cognitively impaired, and presumably would require greater input from care staff, since higher levels of cognitive impairment were also associated with higher levels of dependency. This outcome would appear to concur with that of an American study (Quinn et al., 1999) and a recent UK study (Netten et al., 2001a), which also found an increased prevalence of cognitive impairment in care home residents compared with studies conducted a decade earlier.

Many of the study residents were rated by staff as moderately or severely confused using the Crichton Royal Confusion Subscale, and using the accepted cut points for the Mini Mental State Examination (MMSE), nearly two-thirds (63 per cent) were severely or very severely cognitively impaired. Quinn et al. (1999) found that 60 per cent of residents exhibited some cognitive impairment.

The present study demonstrated the importance in research of involving as many residents as possible regardless of cognitive impairment, since fewer than 5 per cent were unable to complete the MMSE, and just 15 per cent were unable to complete the Geriatric Depression Scale. In fact almost 70 per cent of residents attempted the LQOLP-R and of those, over three-quarters (77.5 per cent) of the interviews were adjudged reliable. In essence, the study found that a minimum level of orientation to place, language and attention was essential for interviewability. This suggests more precise criteria are required for the inclusion of older people for interview than are commonly used.

There were minimal changes in MMSE scores for survivors over time. There were no differences in MMSE scores on entry to the home between those that died and those that survived. However, those who survived had less cognitive decline after admission compared with those who died before the end of the study period.

Quality of life

The findings of this study suggest that activity or occupation is an important aspect of quality of life in care homes. Previous studies conducted with residents of care homes have found that having something meaningful to do is an important part of quality of life (Ball et al., 2000), yet observation studies have reported lack of activity generally in nursing homes (Clark and Bowling, 1990) which is consistent with this study. A positive outcome of one piece of research on the activity needs of care home residents has been the employment of 'leisure therapists' and services specifically tailored to residents' needs (Raynes, 1998).

In this present study, as described in Chapter 4, there were relatively low ratios of care staff to residents in all homes. It is unrealistic under these circumstances to expect care staff to take on the development of activities as part of their responsibilities, since these will inevitably receive lower priority than basic resident care. The creation of dedicated staff for activity may be the only means of ring-fencing time to ensure that it takes place. It is also possible that particular skills are required for effective engagement in activities with people who have severe mental and physical impairments, and the role of specialist staff, such as occupational therapists, in this is worthy of further exploration.

Overall, there was little variation in satisfaction in the quality of life domains for residents who survived over the nine-month study period. Although older generations tend to complain less about situations with which they are not happy (Allen et al., 1992), it is possible that a more sensitive measure of quality of life would be required to detect any changes in satisfaction. A study measuring resident satisfaction with assisted living facilities found a high correlation between resident satisfaction and the Affect Balance Scale, suggesting that satisfaction may be a measure of psychological well-being rather than quality of care (Sikorska-Simmons, 2001).

Satisfaction with health was related to survival, and satisfaction with health at nine months (time 3) was associated with depression at nine months (time 3) and with a measure of the physical comfort of the home. Thus the care environment of the home as measured by the comfort of the surroundings was significantly associated with residents' satisfaction with their health. It is also noteworthy that depression at nine months was predicted by residents' levels of satisfaction with pleasure from things done in the home and with a lack of opportunities for keeping themselves occupied measured at five months (time 2).

A research study of nursing and residential homes for people with dementia (Tune and Bowie, 2000) found that private sector homes provided fewer recreational facilities and were less resident-orientated than public sector homes although the latter were in a poorer physical condition. The authors concluded that the homes could do more at little cost to improve the care environments of the homes. In this present study the outcome of being satisfied with the prospect of living in the home for a long time was related to (lack of) depression at nine months and living in a *positive* or 'Cluster 3' home. Indeed, there was a fair measure of agreement between residents and researchers about whether or not a home was a good one. This was a home in which, according to the staff, there was high *cohesion* (staff are helpful to residents and residents are helpful to each other) and low *conflict* (residents express little anger and little criticism of the home or other residents). These *positive* homes, as described in Chapter 7, were ones in which staff judged the level of work demands, role conflict and job satisfaction to be moderate; and in which they thought there was a working climate which required high effort — significantly higher than in homes in the other two clusters. These homes which both residents and researchers seem to have regarded as good ones did not differ from the others in size or type of home, staff ratio, costs, occupancy levels or the dependency needs of the resident population generally. They were homes in which the staff seem to have been expected to put more energy into their work.

Similarly, a quality of life study conducted with older people in assisted living facilities found high *cohesion* and low *conflict* to be positively correlated with life satisfaction and satisfaction with the facility, and negatively correlated with depression (Mitchell and Kemp, 2000). Regression analyses revealed that facility satisfaction was predicted by high *cohesion* and low *conflict* and fewer chronic health problems. Life satisfaction was predicted by higher *cohesion*, fewer chronic health problems and involvement in social activities and family contact. The authors describe the social climate as the 'personality' of a home, which represents how the resident experiences this environment. They suggest that the social climate of residents' lives contributes most to positive quality of life. Since this plays such a central part in their quality of life, they recommend the building of (in American terms) smaller facilities, the development of training and education programmes that focus on the social environment, and an emphasis on positive resident-staff interactions.

Staff

As discussed in Chapter 6, staff members made a very significant contribution to the care environment. Although fewer staff returned questionnaires than had been hoped, analysis of the data revealed some interesting findings about staff training and their level of knowledge of residents in their care, as well as on their pay and employment conditions.

Returned questionnaires revealed a lack of basic training for both nursing and care assistants in their current job, in particular training in the care and management of dementia and depression, psychiatric or psychological problems generally, and in the emotional care of residents. In fact, few of the care staff who returned questionnaires had received training on depression or mental health in their current job despite an average duration of 4.2 years in post. Staff training was not seen as a priority in most of the homes. The requirements set out in the National Minimum Standards for Care Homes (Department of Health, 2001a) that half of all care staff should attain NVQ level 2 by 2005, may go some way to address this. However the cost of training care staff, both in terms of time and money, will be an important consideration in the outcome of this standard (Bagley et al., 2002).

In addition to mental health, medication represents another area where there is need for increased training input. The high rate of prescription medication for residents and the effects of polypharmacy as discussed earlier in this chapter, have implications not only for residents in terms of better access to primary care, but also for the training of staff in basic awareness of potential medication problems. The *National Service Framework for Older People* document, *Medicines and Older People* (Department of Health, 2001c) sets out a number of recommendations relating to these aspects of care.

In addition to the work of Moxon et al. (2001) described above, two training programmes for care staff have been reported, whose outcomes have met with mixed success. The first dealt with problem behaviour in residents (Moniz-Cook et al., 1998) and the second was undertaken to improve quality of staff/ patient interactions (Proctor et al., 1998). In the first, following training using a person-centred approach to dementia care, care staff reported less difficulty in managing problem behaviour although the frequencies of behaviour did not change. However, the effects of the programme were not long-lasting and it was suggested that regular consultation sessions or more specialised interventions may be required. In the second, a multidisciplinary old age psychiatry team delivered training seminars which covered the physical and mental health of older people and the value of activities. At the end of the training period levels of resident activity had increased and there was an improvement in staff-resident interactions. In this present study, home managers reported that based on the total population of their homes, an average of 14 per cent of residential home and 25 per cent of nursing home residents had behavioural problems, with a great deal of variation between homes. There was also little evidence of resident activity or verbal contact between staff and residents. Thus, training to improve knowledge of the care of older people, or to deal with problem behaviours may have some benefits in helping staff with their caring role and in improving residents' relationships and levels of activity.

Nurses failed to recognise depressive symptoms in residents on entry to the homes in two-thirds of cases and their recognition rates were similar to staff without formal nurse training. The value that the Royal College of Nursing places on the specific abilities of nurses as skilled practitioners (Royal College of Nursing, 1997), particularly in the context of conducting assessments with older people, indicates that specific training in the recognition of depression in older people is required. Indeed, research has established a positive association between overall educational preparation of nursing staff in nursing homes and quality of care, as indicated by a measure of resident autonomy (Davies et al., 1999). A survey of student placements in nursing homes found that, on the whole, placements were a positive experience for nursing students. Those who did not enjoy the placement were able to recognise its value at a later stage. Matrons and staff alike recognised the role of students in raising the profile of nursing home care (Wade and Skinner, 2001). Thus, developing links between educational centres and nursing homes would be beneficial to residents, staff and nursing students alike. In a survey of old age psychiatry services in England it was found that 47 per cent provided formal training sessions in mental health to residential and nursing homes (Challis et al., 2002b). However, no data were available on the extent of coverage, and the proportion of homes in an area which had access was not known. Given that slightly less than half of services provide this level of support, it would appear that this is a means whereby skills in the recognition of, and responses to mental health problems might be improved. In the US, the teaching nursing home has developed as a model centre of excellence and similar initiatives could be of value in the UK (Lipsitz, 1994).

Research conducted in nursing homes in Sweden involved training care staff in the use of a standardised assessment, the Minimum Data Set/Resident Assessment Instrument (MDS/RAI) (Morris et al., 1990). One year later a majority of staff agreed that it had improved quality of care in terms of information and knowledge about the residents, staff observational ability and care planning, although assessments were time consuming. It was also seen as beneficial in facilitating relationships with relatives by actively involving them in the assessment process (Hansebo et al., 1998).

It would seem, therefore, that in order to improve the situation for residents in terms of better recognition of mental health problems, rehabilitation, reduction in dependency and encouragement to take part in activities inside and outside the home, it is important that care staff be regarded as a central part of the care environment. The potentially important contribution of closer links with old age psychiatry services has already been noted. This could have the effect of bringing new ideas into homes and of reducing the potential insular experience of staff working in isolation. The lack of preparation for their role, inferior conditions of employment, and experience of isolation from both residents and the wider community has been acknowledged by others (Davies, 2001). The cost in terms of time and money to provide training, and improvements in the pay and conditions for some care staff could help to improve the social care workforce overall and would, no doubt, benefit the residents of care homes in the long run (Department of Health, 2000).

Relatives' satisfaction

Although the concern to make services more responsive to the needs of carers has tended to focus on home-based care, carer well-being can be significantly influenced by the quality of care provided by a care home (Challis and Davies, 1986; Wells and Jorm, 1987; Gilleard 1992; Levin et al., 1994). There is evidence of this particularly in homes where efforts are made to assist family carers in continuing their caring role to a certain degree (Moriarty and Webb, 2000). However other research conducted with the relatives of older people living in nursing homes found that relatives were unhappy with the amount of time staff had to talk to them, felt staff lacked knowledge about the residents, and that relatives desired better communication and involvement with staff (Hertzberg and Ekman 2000; Ryan and Scullion, 2000; Hertzberg et al., 2001).

In this present study, just over two-thirds (68 per cent) of relatives who returned a questionnaire had received information about the care home, and of this group, a similar proportion (70 per cent) were happy with the standard of the information they received. The need for care homes to produce information booklets describing the home and its ethos has been set out in *Fit For The Future* (Department of Health, 1999). This consultation document undertaken by the Centre for Policy on Ageing, suggested that homes should make clear their style and philosophy of care through a brochure or prospectus. This was confirmed as Standard 1 in the National Minimum Standards in Care Homes for Older People (Department of Health, 2001a).

As described in Chapter 8, a number of questionnaires returned by the relatives included comments about the building and accommodation, activities and social opportunities in the home, and the care received by the residents. Some of these individual comments were negative or critical of the home, in particular in relation to meals, room sharing and room size, home facilities, standards of furniture and equipment, and residents' clothing and appearance. It is noteworthy that a number of these criteria are identified in the National Minimum Care Standards in Care Homes for Older People (Department of Health, 2001a).

So what makes a good care home?

The outcome of living in a care home might be considered to be related to two factors, namely the mental and physical well-being of residents at entry (their level of needs), and the processes of care within the home. It is clearly important to take account of both factors (Kane et al., 1983; Kane and Kane, 1987; Mor, 2003) and both were addressed in the analyses described in Chapter 11. A key question identified in Chapter 1 was whether a better resident outcome was more likely in some homes than others. This is reviewed here.

A home in which residents have plenty to do?

Of overwhelming importance in determining length of survival or nine-month outcome were the individual characteristics residents brought with them to the home — notably the level of dependency as measured by the Barthel. The differential effects of aspects of the care environment were harder to detect. However this study provides, possibly for the first time, evidence of the influence of opportunities for occupation and pleasure in the home. These appear to be significant contributors both to survival and to mood state nine months after admission. Residents who obtained little pleasure from things they did in the home were more likely to die and more likely to be depressed after nine months. This observation should be viewed in the light of other findings from this study. It may be recalled that one-third of residents questioned shortly after admission were dissatisfied with the provision of occupational opportunities. Based on 2001 figures (Department of Health, 2001e) there may be, in nursing and residential homes in England alone, about 125,000 elderly people who agree with them.

In the present study, of 5400 observations of residents in 'public space' 51 per cent were of residents sitting in complete inactivity, either awake or dozing in their chairs. In 80 per cent of the study homes there was less than six minutes of activity staff time available, per occupied bed, per day. A study of seventeen care facilities for people with dementia, using Dementia Care Mapping (Ballard et al., 2001b) found similarly disheartening results. Over a six hour period of daytime observation, residents spent nearly one-third of their time socially withdrawn or inactive (30 per cent). Just 50 minutes of their day was spent in communication with staff or other residents, (14 per cent), and less than 12 minutes (3 per cent) was spent in constructive activity other than watching TV. The authors recommend the review and improvement of standards in care homes and draw attention to the key domain of interaction and daily activity as set out in the National Care Standards (Department of Health, 2001a).

The picture that appears to emerge is that in the main, residents of care homes are generally inactive and isolated from each other in some degree. It has been reported that older people experience social isolation as a result of admission to a long-stay care home (Royal Commission on Long Term Care, 1999) and that nursing homes are also isolated from the communities in which they are placed (Davies, 2001). In fact, the term 'islands of the old' has been coined as a metaphor for care homes (Reed, 1998), and further described by Davies (2001) as appropriate in view of the little contact residents and care staff have with their local community. When these points are considered together they make a strong case for putting resources into improving the quality and quantity of occupational opportunities for care home residents, and for providing services which help them remain in contact with 'the outside world', or encourage the integration of the home into the local community (Reed et al., 1998, Department of Health, 1999; 2001a)

A home with low conflict and high cohesion?

It is noteworthy that there was a fair measure of agreement between residents and researchers regarding 'good' homes, that is homes where residents were happier about the prospect of remaining. These were ones in which the Sheltered Care Environment Scale, completed by staff, showed low scores for *conflict* (extent to which residents express anger or criticise each other or the home) and high ones for *cohesion* (extent of helpfulness of staff to residents and between residents). This was not related to physical characteristics of the building nor to factors such as the staff ratio. It was related to whether staff perceived the workplace as being one in which they were expected to put extra effort into their work.

An association between resident satisfaction with a care home and staff attitudes or helpfulness has been found in a number of studies (Grau et al., 1995; Ball et al., 2000). In a study carried out in the Netherlands, nursing home residents were asked whether they 'felt at home' in the nursing home (de Veer and Kerkstra, 2001). 'Feeling at home' was related to resident-centredness and disturbance caused by other residents. Resident-centredness described homes where residents were treated with respect and kindness, had someone to confide in and someone who showed an interest in the resident and their life history. Residents who did not feel at home mentioned the attitudes of nurses more often and judged the staff as less resident-centred.

Components of a good home?

If it were possible to combine together the findings of this chapter thus far, and assuming that survival is one of the valued outcomes, then a good home provides: satisfaction with pleasure from things done in the home; forms of chosen and appropriate valued activity; opportunities for keeping occupied in the home; staff working in a cohesive fashion; little conflict; and finally good physical comfort. These are summarised in Box 12.1.

Environment and outcomes

This list of care environment characteristics which had an effect on outcome for care home residents, is a short one. Nevertheless, it does identify some improvements to which home providers, purchasers and inspectors might aspire. The first involves a clear plan of action, albeit one which is not without cost. Over a number of years researchers have commented on the general level

---

Box 12.1
Qualities of a good home

A good quality care home provides residents with:
- opportunities for keeping occupied in the home
- activities that are appropriate and valued
- satisfaction with pleasure from things done in the home
- staff working cohesively
- lack of conflict
- good physical comfort

---

of inactivity in UK homes (for example Godlove et al., 1982; Willcocks et al., 1987; Clark and Bowling, 1990). A brief passage from the report of an American study serves to illustrate how differently the baseline level of provision is seen in some other countries: 'From a large nursing care facility, 60 elderly patients diagnosed as having Alzheimer's disease were randomly separated into three groups of equal size ... For music Group 1 'Big Band' music from the 1920s and 1930s was played during their daily recreation period while Group 2 were given puzzle exercises during their activity sessions. Members of Group 3 participated in the *standard recreational activities of drawing and painting.*' (Lord and Garner, 1993) (our italics). Such activities are far from being 'standard' in homes in the UK. This study now provides evidence that better provision of occupational opportunities — helping residents to get more pleasure out of their daily lives in care homes — may have real benefits in improved outcome. Given the severe mental and physical disabilities of many residents this is unlikely to happen without employment of skilled staff. It takes dedicated time, skill and perseverance to help people who may be depressed and demotivated find occupations that are meaningful to them. Whether this service is directly delivered by qualified staff, or by assistants supervised by qualified staff working in a number of homes, this could, for example, be provided by occupational therapists.

The second link found between care environment and outcome is less easy to act upon. A simple recommendation that care home providers, purchasers and inspectors should aim for homes with low *conflict* and high *cohesion* scores on the Sheltered Care Environment Scale (SCES) is unlikely to be viewed as helpful. However it may be helpful at least to contemplate this as one way of understanding the features of care homes which contribute to good resident outcomes. Ways may be found to use the SCES in inspection processes (though this is not without obvious difficulties). For example, it provides domains to focus upon and observe, namely conflict and cohesion. Alternatively, it could be used as the basis for staff training or discussions between residents and staff.

Balancing risk and opportunities in care settings

In recent years social commentators, researchers and policy makers have become more aware of the need to permit (or even legislate for) greater autonomy, independence and control for older people living in long-stay care homes. Nevertheless, there is still much debate regarding how best to balance the rights of residents on the one hand, with the issue of safety on the other, while maintaining best possible quality of life. In the US, evidence of poor nursing home care throughout the 1970s resulted in the introduction of the Omnibus Budget Reconciliation Act 1987 (OBRA 87). This Act created a set of minimum standards of care and rights for people living in Medicare or Medicaid long-term care facilities. It required homes to emphasise resident quality of life as well as quality of care; maintain or improve residents' activities of daily living; employ trained and certified aides; and apply strict guidelines to the use of medication and physical restraints (Turnham, 2001). Subsequent improvements have been reported by a number of commentators in the quality of care of home residents in the US (Phillips et al., 1996; Lacey, 1999; Kane, 2001).

The introduction of the Minimum Data Set (MDS) (Morris et al., 1990) as part of these changes in America has allowed quality indicators to be measured across care homes. However it is important that there is a balance between resident choice and autonomy and care outcomes. For example, a desire to reduce the number of resident falls should not impose excessive restrictions upon the residents. Kane (2001) argues that the goals set by health regulators and policymakers may force clients into more protected settings, compromising residents' quality of life, and challenges the assumption that safety is the most important factor in the long-term care of older people. She believes that older people may prefer the 'best health and safety outcomes possible *that are consistent with a meaningful quality of life* ...' rather than, 'the best quality of life *as is consistent with health and safety*.' (her italics).

In the UK it has been suggested that quality of life in residential care is influenced to a large extent by the attitudes of owners and the quality of staff at all levels (Norman, 1980; Centre for Policy on Ageing, 1984). The balance between quality of life and risk of accidents is illustrated in a study that compared long-stay hospital care and NHS nursing home care (Bowling et al., 1992). It found that the nursing home environment was more flexible although the risk of accidents was far higher. However individuals in the hospital setting had a poorer quality of life. The authors concluded that care home staff should accept the degree of risk and take preventative steps to ensure a safer physical environment. The Centre for Policy on Ageing report *Home Life* (CPA, 1984) considered 'responsible risk-taking' one of a number of concepts that formed the basis for good residential care practice. It recommended that residents should not be denied certain activities purely on the grounds that some degree of risk was involved.

Those who wish to see more choice and autonomy for residents in care homes are happy to accept that risk is a normal part of adult life. In particular, the 'Eden Alternative'™ (Thomas, 1994; 1996) developed in America to transform the nursing home environment by the introduction of plants, pets and young people, does by its very nature involve risks to staff and residents. However, understanding and minimising these risks by careful planning may reduce the risk of accidents or injuries (Barba et al., 2002). Interestingly, such approaches are not new, and similar features to the 'Eden Alternative' may be found in the principles of mental health care developed by the Tukes at the Retreat in York (Tuke, 1813, reprinted 1996). Nevertheless, there has been evidence of positive changes in residents' perceptions of control over their daily lives and satisfaction with nursing care in homes incorporating the 'Eden Alternative' (Drew and Brooke, 1999).

On a similar theme, a survey of long-term care facilities providing outdoor areas found them to be beneficial and provide stimulation to residents. However, due to fears about their safety, these areas were not used as much as they could be (Cohen-Mansfield and Werner, 1999). Outdoor activities included eating and barbecues, exercise, parties and gardening, yet while there were obvious benefits for cognitively impaired residents and 'wanderers', many facilities encountered problems relating to the safety of residents, and with regard to demands on staff time and attention. The authors describe a number of potential safety features available and maintain that it is possible to improve resident well-being with the use of outdoor areas without endangering their safety.

It has been argued that residents should be regarded as 'partners', active in the care process, rather than passive recipients of care, such that care staff are regarded less as guardians, and the issues of independence and safety are more balanced between staff and residents (Booth, 1985; Davies, 2001). It is perhaps not surprising that the issue of safety is a concern for care providers more than residents. In a recent study of resident quality of life in assisted living facilities, both providers and residents tended to mention fairly similar domains as important to resident quality of life but resident safety and well-being was more of an overriding concern for care providers (Ball et al., 2000). Although the authors acknowledged that residents desired independence and autonomy, providers faced particular ethical dilemmas in striking the correct balance. One answer, they suggest, could be simply to increase the level of staffing. Kane (2001) believes that it is important that care home owners who are willing to accept some negotiated risks are not penalised for 'untoward events', thus encouraging the withdrawal of activities and autonomy beneficial to those living in long-term care.

Thus, the relationship between the physical and social environment, quality of life and resident security, safety, psychological well-being and quality of care is a complex one, involving trade-offs between different domains. Activity, identified in this study as important, depends upon the capacity of staff to evaluate and manage risk so as to permit a degree of resident autonomy.

Implications for policy

This study has identified a number of policy issues in relation to care homes for older people. Its organising theme was entirely in line with the prevailing concern with quality (Department of Health, 2000). Indeed the study was designed to examine quality of life and its determinants in the content of quality of services and care environments. As discussed in Chapter 1, quality may be observed in the outcomes of care, the ways in which needs are identified and the content of the care provided. The 'Quality Strategy' developed by the UK government in the field of social care (Department of Health, 2000) builds upon the themes in the White Paper *Modernising Social Services* (Cm 4169, 1998). It focuses upon the three tasks of enhancing the consistency of social services, creating more accessible and individually tailored services, and enhancing the skills and competencies of the workforce. Related to these are the specific developments of more systematic approaches to assessment of older people through the Single Assessment Process (SAP) (Department of Health, 2002a), and to rehabilitation and Intermediate Care (Department of Health, 2001d; Steiner, 2001).

The policy issues highlighted by this study can be summarised as related to quality, both in terms of identification of resident perceptions of quality and of staff skills; assessment; and the content of care. Each of these is discussed briefly below.

Quality issues

Ascertaining older people's views about quality of service The study findings suggest that many older people are capable, even in the presence of significant cognitive impairment, of answering questions about their quality of life and satisfaction with services. This is relevant to the quality assurance strategies to be developed using consumer satisfaction as an evaluative criterion (Cm 4169, 1998). Accordingly, it would seem reasonable that research concerning the health and well-being of older people, and all service evaluations, including evaluation of user satisfaction, should make strenuous efforts to be as inclusive as possible, and should use, and report, rational criteria for any exclusions of individuals for reasons such as cognitive impairment (Mozley et al., 1999).

This has been given particular salience in recent policy developments. Despite the introduction of the Care Standards Act (2000) and the establishment of the National Minimum Care Standards (Department of Health, 2001a), some commentators have been critical of the lack of accountability given to service users (Kerrison and Pollock, 2001a). Although *Fit for the Future* (Department of Health, 1999) was a joint effort involving different agencies, standards have already been vulnerable to industry lobbying, particularly with regard to minimum room sizes and changes to staffing ratios (Department of Health, 2002b). The authors conclude that the lack of emphasis on service user involvement or rights means that the private health care sector is being treated differently from other consumer sectors. While the reasons for this may be economic, they may also be cultural, since until recently, users of public services such as the NHS had no rights in terms of the decision-making process and few rights to complain (Kerrison and Pollock, 2001b). However, the present study has indicated that valid opinions about quality of care may be obtained from vulnerable older people. The study also produces recommendations for some of the questions that might be included in service evaluation exercises. Four indicators were found to be of particular value: residents' assessments of satisfaction with their own health; with the pleasure they got from things they did in the home; with the occupational opportunities available; and with the prospect of living in the home for a long time. The last of these four questions is commended to researchers as a good indicator of overall satisfaction with a home and its services.

Staff Recent policy initiatives have stressed the importance of the workforce as part of the new quality agenda (Department of Health, 2000). Specific targets have been announced regarding the training of staff working in care homes. Under the new regulatory framework, the training of care staff must be accredited and include basic knowledge of how medicines are used and how to recognise and deal with problems in their use (Department of Health, 2001a). Furthermore, all staff are expected to complete a comprehensive induction programme in their first six weeks of employment with further training to be given within the first six months of employment. Apart from the manager of the home, there must be a minimum of 50 per cent of the staff including agency staff, in residential homes qualified to NVQ Level 2 or its equivalent by 2005. In nursing homes, apart from one-third of the staff being registered nurses, the remaining care staff would require the same proportion qualified to NVQ Level 2 (Department of Health, 1999; 2001a). Staff should receive a minimum of three paid days' training per year, and have an individual training and development assessment (Department of Health, 2001a). However, the extent to which these targets will be attained has been questioned (O'Kell, 2002). Appropriate training materials are likely to be required to address specific aspects of need such as depression or dementia (Bhaduri, 2001).

The *National Service Framework for Older People* (NSFOP) noted that specialist mental health services should provide training and advice for professionals and other staff whose responsibilities include providing care and treatment for older people with mental health problems, including those working in residential and nursing home care (Department of Health, 2001b: 7.54, 7.56). This was endorsed by the Audit Commission (2002). However, specialist mental health services are varied in their pattern of working and in England less than 50 per cent of old age psychiatry services worked to improve early recognition of mental health problems or provided training to care home staff (Challis et al., 2002b). Glendinning et al. (2002) found that direct access to old age psychiatry services was only available to just over 10 per cent of homes and up to 10 per cent of homes had no old age psychiatrist available to visit when required.

It is interesting to consider whether these training requirements will equip care staff with greater competence to do the job and a better understanding of residents' needs. Conceivably this could contribute to job satisfaction and constitute a modest step towards addressing factors associated with staff turnover such as the low prestige and lack of career structure of long-term care work. Many of the staff in this study were poorly paid and lacked occupational pensions. Labour market conditions have made the care sector relatively unattractive as an employment option, with wider opportunities and greater remuneration in the commercial sector (O'Kell, 2002). However, O'Kell (2002) identified staff retention as more likely in homes that assist staff to take up education and training opportunities. Nevertheless, greater recognition through training is unlikely to contribute to recruitment and retention alone, without the relative pay, conditions and career prospects of care workers being enhanced.

Assessment

Two aspects of assessment are relevant to the study's findings. The first relates to assessment prior to entry, used as a means to ensure that people who enter care homes are those for whom it is most beneficial. The second relates to the nature of assessment processes within care homes, which may contribute to better identification of the needs of residents and lead to better care.

Pre-admission assessment and advice This study demonstrated that many of the older people who were admitted to nursing homes had low dependency needs. This was particularly so with regard to self-funding residents. A national study has confirmed this picture of better physical functioning and lower cognitive impairment in self-funded compared with publicly funded residents, particularly in residential homes (Netten et al., 2001c).

There is a substantial literature on the benefits of systematic assessment prior to care home admission. Brocklehurst et al. (1978) and Sharma et al. (1994) found significant minorities of residents who did not need that level of care. Most countries are pursuing policies of downward substitution, to avoid inappropriate high cost care solutions wherever possible. In both the US and Switzerland comprehensive geriatric assessment has been associated with a reduction in the risk of nursing home placement (Applegate et al., 1990; Stuck et al., 1995).

This present study has identified that some inappropriate placement still appears to occur. It supports the conclusion that the pursuit of residential independence for frail older people, emphasised in a range of policies from the late 1980s (Cm849, 1989) through more recent documents (Cm 4169, 1998) and the NSFOP (Department of Health, 2001b), requires full multidisciplinary assessment of physical and mental health and a full medication review. Current policy is concerned to develop greater consistency in approaches to care (Cm 4169, 1998), through a variety of mechanisms incorporated in the NSFOP (Department of Health, 2001b). That there is considerable variation in recognition of major needs is clearly contrary to this.

The Care Standards Act (2000) has specified the importance of a pre-admission home assessment by staff. In the National Minimum Standards for Care Homes (Department of Health, 2001a), Standard 3 specifies that new residents are only to be admitted to homes on the basis of a full assessment undertaken by people trained to do so. However, these processes vary according to the means of funding of the potential resident.

For those admitted with public funding the SAP (Department of Health, 2002a) provides the means by which that will be undertaken. The SAP constitutes one part of a strategy to reduce inappropriate variation in patterns of care, following evidence of marked variability in assessment processes for older people (Stewart et al., 1999). It was designed to: ensure that older people receive appropriate effective and timely responses to their health and social care needs; ensure that professional resources are used effectively, and produce greater consistency and quality of assessment. Nine domains of assessment are part of the process and a number of assessment tools are listed as exemplars by the Department of Health in the guidance. A comprehensive assessment should be completed for those where levels of support and treatment likely to be offered are intensive or prolonged, including permanent admission to a care home. This is expected to be multidisciplinary and should involve input from geriatricians, old age psychiatrists, registered nurses, allied health professionals, and social workers (Department of Health, 2002a). Home managers should be fully involved in the admission and play an important part in care planning, monitoring and review. For nursing home care, an older person's assessment of needs and care plan must involve a registered nurse employed by NHS who will help determine the setting in which care is to be provided, and determine the appropriate level of Registered Nursing Care Contribution (Department of Health, 2001f) to the funding of their care.

For those who are self-funded the home has to carry out an assessment with 13 specified domains. This part of Standard 3 of the National Minimum Care Standards (Department of Health, 2001a) is designed to ensure that the content of assessment of these residents is more specific than hitherto. However, there remain differences between the assessment domains of the SAP and those within the National Care Standards. The use of more standardised approaches to the assessment and review of residents in care homes is one strategy which could address this issue.

Obviously, the range of personnel and services available in any given locality to contribute to this assessment process will vary. However, the new requirements move considerably closer to that which was adopted in the Australian Aged Care Reforms, which required entry to a nursing or hostel place to take place only after assessment by an Aged Care Assessment Team (Challis et al., 1995; 1998). This has the advantage that it makes for formal links between secondary care services such as geriatric medicine and old age psychiatry and the provision of community based care.

Assessment after admission One of the expectations from a more structured approach to assessment, arising from the SAP (Department of Health, 2002a), would be an improvement in the recognition of important areas of need. However, there is no formal guidance, either as part of the SAP or in the National Minimum Care Standards, as to the form or content of assessment within care homes.

As described in Chapter 1, standardised resident assessment has been a feature of nursing home care in the US for many years. The MDS/RAI (Morris et al., 1990) has been used widely to assess residents on admission and the UK version (Challis et al., 2000a) is an approach cited by the Department of Health for use in care homes (Department of Health, 2002c). Reactions to the RAI from care staff in the US regarding its ability to improve quality have been mixed: some reported that it improved their ability to determine whether care plans were effective, and some have found it time consuming (Hawes et al., 1997). One possible concern about structured approaches, such as the MDS/RAI, is that staff may focus attention on the needs of particular sub-populations of residents, particularly those with the greatest care needs, at the expense of those with less functional dependence. Consequently, efforts to improve areas related to mood and behaviour for all residents may be neglected (Phillips et al., 1997) unless particular managerial effort is made to focus upon these areas of need. The present study has demonstrated the extent to which a key aspect of quality of life, whether or not a person suffered from depression, was frequently missed by all grades of staff in the absence of structured assessment. One solution to the problem of assessment of depression in care homes is the use of a standardised depression measure such as the GDS-12R (Sutcliffe et al., 2000), developed in the present study.

Content of care

Three areas relating to the content of care emerge as relevant from the study. First is the crucial observation that activity provided within the home can make a significant difference. Second is the relationship between the current focus upon rehabilitation and prevention, and the lack of appropriate resources to achieve this in care home settings. Third is the need to consider the development of greater expertise in the care home setting in dealing with mental disorders in older people.

Opportunities for occupation and 'pleasure in the home' The present study indicated the importance of activity as a determinant of certain aspects of quality of life, including the older person's mood state and subjective well-being. It is noteworthy that this was confirmed by studies in the US where activities were associated with lower death rates and less functional decline (Spector and Takada, 1999) and depression was lower in settings where activities were provided (Mitchell and Kemp, 2000). There is definitely scope for further research to investigate the impact on the prevalence of depression in care homes of the introduction of activity programmes. An intervention study to determine if occupational therapy can reduce depression among care home residents, by encouraging participation in activities that develop everyday life skills, is currently under way (Mozley et al., 2003).

Fit for the Future (Department of Health, 1999) produced by the Centre for Policy on Ageing, took account of the fact that residents vary in their desire for involvement in activities or in the social life of a home. However both this and the Audit Commission's *Forget Me Not* (2000a) have recommended the need to maintain opportunities for residents to engage in social activities. The Care Standards Act has formally entrenched this into the regulatory process. The National Minimum Standards for Care Homes for Older People recommend that routines of daily living and activities should be flexible and varied to suit residents' expectations, preferences and capacities. Residents' interests should be recorded and they should be given opportunities for leisure and recreational activities both within and outside the home which suit their needs, including access to and use of gardens (Department of Health, 2001a). The balancing of risk with care is also acknowledged in the recognition that some individuals may want the capacity to play an active part in food preparation. Since access to kitchens may compromise health and safety considerations, homes are expected to examine alternative ways of maintaining residents' involvement such as providing kitchenettes, organising cooking as part of a range of daily activities and enabling residents to help in the dining room (Department of Health, 2001a). Others, however, may equally desire privacy and independence. Thus the application of the standards and the regime in the homes will have to respond to this wide variation in preferences. Furthermore, regulations give residents the opportunity to have a say in how the social life of the home is run (Department of Health, 1999; Department of Health, 2001a).

The importance of activities shown by the present study reinforces the significance of these requirements and a range of opportunities for occupation and entertainment are likely to be required. It would seem logical that homes should be required to employ dedicated staff for this purpose and provide an activities budget. However, it is likely that remuneration rates for care will need to take this additional service requirement into account. Currently there are closures of care homes (Netten et al., 2002), with some 12,600 places lost during 2001 (Laing and Buisson, 2001). Furthermore, current public funding is estimated to be insufficient for the provision of care at a suitable standard or to encourage investment in good quality new nursing home stock (Laing, 1998). In one study 60 per cent of home closures were attributed to the requirements of the care standards (Netten et al., 2002).

Rehabilitation Policy guidance has stressed the importance of rehabilitation in the care of older people (Department of Health, 1997). More recently, the intro-duction of Intermediate Care (Cm 4818-1, 2000; Department of Health 2001a,d) and the preventative agenda (Cm 4169, 1998) have rendered rehabilitation activities more significant. The need for homes to have access to specialist ser-vices and expertise to manage problems such as incontinence more effectively has been noted elsewhere (Peet et al., 1994). The lack of activity and of therapy services noted in the present study is therefore particularly pertinent.

There is clear evidence of marked variation in access to specialist services by care homes (Jacobs et al., 2001). Jacobs and Rummery (2002) conclude that shortfalls in the provision of NHS services to nursing homes may hinder the rehabilitation potential of intermediate care placements in nursing homes. Thus, although the Audit Commission (Audit Commission, 2000b) has indi-cated that good assessment and multidisciplinary rehabilitation could reduce the risk of hospital admission or readmission for older people, lack of access to such services in homes could increase the risk of unnecessary admission and disrupt the continuity of care.

Effective approaches to rehabilitation and prevention in the widest sense can only occur in care homes where the standards of assessment are significantly improved and where the external inputs of expertise to facilitate caring for vulnerable older people are arranged on a more systematic basis than currently. There will be a need to detect presence of conditions requiring intervention which is dependent upon improved assessment, which may itself in part depend upon external expertise. There is clearly a need to ensure that homes have access to specialist skills to a less variable extent than at present. For example, Standard 8 of the National Care Standards aims to ensure that: service users' health care needs are fully met; opportunities are given for appropriate exercise and physical activity; and service users are given access to NHS services by providing them with information about entitlements and facilitating their access to appropriate advice (Department of Health, 2001a). This will require less variability in access to primary care (Glendinning et al., 2002), specialist services (Jacobs et al., 2001) and extended roles for old age psychiatry and geriatric medicine in relation to care homes (Black and Bowman, 1997; Challis et al., 1998; 2002b).

Effective care for residents with mental health problems It has already been noted that recognition of depression in care homes, by qualified nurses as well as by unqualified staff, was poor. There is need to address this significant staff training issue, in the context not only of in-service training but also of nursing education. Depression appears to affect a very high proportion of care home residents (Mann et al., 1984; 2000) and routine screening as part of regular health checks might be one way to ensure that adequate diagnosis and treatment are provided by mental health specialists.

The study also demonstrated that people with significant cognitive impairment are admitted to both residential and nursing homes. As a consequence, the care of people with dementia cannot be regarded only as a special need for which only a minority of homes need to cater. It is, for a significant proportion of residents, a major reason for admission (Netten et al., 2001a, b; Macdonald et al., 2002). *All* care homes therefore need to be designed, operated and staffed with this in mind.

With regard to residents with considerable cognitive impairment, a Dementia Care Mapping study of residents with dementia (Bruce et al., 2002) found that some care environments were less able to meet the complex needs of residents with severe impairment, in contrast to those who were less impaired with less complex needs. The former tended to be less predictable, less able to communicate or less responsive and thus staff concentrated their efforts on residents who were more rewarding. Residents with low 'well-being' had their physical needs attended to satisfactorily. However, this left little time for their social, emotional or occupational needs. The authors suggest that care staff require particular skills to meet the needs of more disabled residents who are less rewarding to care for, ongoing support and guidance to develop these skills, and need to be shown that their efforts to care for residents with more complex needs are worthwhile.

Indeed, the Audit Commission recommends that agencies should ensure that there is sufficient residential and nursing home care of good quality available for older people with mental health problems including some specialist provision (Audit Commission, 2002). In addition, specialist services should review their local arrangements for training and supporting GPs and primary care teams in the diagnosis and management of dementia and depression where appropriate (Audit Commission 2000a; 2002).

If both the requirements for more consistency in care services and for access for older people in care homes to specialist mental health services are to be met, considerable change in the pattern of work in old age psychiatry services will be required. This would involve a greater degree of outreach and training by specialist services for care home staff than is currently the case (Challis et al., 2002b).

In conclusion

No claim must be made that this study has succeeded in distilling in full the essence of what it is to provide good quality care. The fact that some expected features of a good quality care home were not identified as significant does not mean they are unimportant — merely that over nine months they did not produce effects sufficiently large to be observable using the particular measures chosen, or that they are closely correlated with those predictors listed. It is possible that if this study had continued to follow the cohort residents to their deaths, other factors would have emerged. It is also possible that different, or more sensitive, measures would have shown larger effects.

One final possibility must be mentioned. It may be that, once care is provided at least above some minimum baseline, differences in ethos or care practice between homes have little effect on residents, and the physical and mental disabilities of individual residents, coupled with the impact of residence in a home — any home — overwhelm in importance any differences in care unless they are very extreme. If that is so, the study's findings on the effects of occupation and 'pleasure in the home' stand out in high relief.

The list of key determinants of quality of life in care homes is a short one. But it does exist. The conclusion to this study is not the fatalistic one that nothing appears to make very much difference. Quite a lot of things appear to make no difference — at least over the period of nine months. But that aspects of a 'good home' can be identified, and that 'pleasure in the home' and opportunities to be occupied make a difference in terms of the probability of death or depression, are significant findings that call for action.

Appendix 1: Observation Study Method

Reproduced from documents used in the study (pages have been reduced in size for this volume).

OBSERVATION STUDY METHOD

This is a variation on the method used by Lemke and Moos (1984).

In each study home eight observational 'sweeps' of the building will be done, starting on the hour between 10am and 5pm. No more than 4 'sweeps' should be done in any one home on the same day. The 'sweeps' will take varying lengths of time depending on the size and complexity of the building. Tour the whole building, ignoring all closed doors and private rooms (even with doors open); also all bathrooms etc.

Using a Psion organiser spreadsheet (set up as described below) twelve variables will be recorded for each resident seen in 'public' space, recording data for each resident on a separate spreadsheet row. Of these twelve variables only the last five will vary between individual residents; the first seven are variables which identify the home, the observer and the observation session and entries will therefore be identical for all residents observed during that particular session.

Setting up the Psion Spreadsheet

On a spreadsheet file enter the twelve variable names below along the top row in columns A1-L1. Enter the additional column heading 'Comments' on the top row of column M1. Using the 'Titles On' facility in the View Menu set the variable names as titles so that they remain in view when scrolling down below row 9. Also using the View Menu increase the width of Column M to 30 characters.

Spreadsheet code column letter	Variable name	Variable description	Value
A	HOMID	Home ID number	
B	OBSRID	Observer ID number	
C	TYPEOB 1....ordinary 2....reliability	Type of observation	

D	MONTHOB 1....January	Month of observation	
	2....February		
	3....March		
E	DAYOB 1....Monday	Day of observation	
	2....Tuesday		
	3.....Weds		
	4....Thursday		
	5....Friday		
	6....Saturday		
	7....Sunday		
F	TIMEOB	Time of observation start	10....10 am 11....11 am 12....12 noon 13....1 pm etc.
G	BEDSOCC	Number of occupied beds in the home on observation day	
H	LOCATION	Location of resident	1....hallway 2....lounge 3....dining room 4....outside 5....other 'public' space

I	ACTIVITY	Activity of resident	1....sleeping / dozing 2....awake 3....performing self- care activities 4....listening to radio / watching TV (with apparent attention) 5....independent pursuit 6....chores 7....group activity 8....locomotion 9....undirected activity 10...eating / drinking 11...other / uncodable
J	VERBAL	Verbal activity of resident	0...silent 1...quiet speech 2...loud speech 3...being spoken to 4...noise 5...conversation 6...other
K	STAFF1	Staff contact first	0....no staff contact 1....nurse / sister / matron 2....nursing asst/carer 3....'other' in house staff 4....visiting professional
L	STAFF2	Staff contact second	0....no staff contact 1....nurse / sister / matron 2....nursing asst/carer 3....'other' in house staff 4....visiting professional
M	COMMENTS	30 character width column for entry of brief note on	any unusual or uncodable behaviours

Recording data on the Psion spreadsheet

Enter data to identify the home, the observer and the observation session in variables A - G inclusive.

Begin observation tour by entering data for the first resident observed along the same row as the variable A - G 'home level' data described above.

For all subsequent residents seen in that observation session use cursor to move between spreadsheet columns H I J K L, leaving A - G blank. Add occasional comments in Column M as and when necessary.

At end of observation session, enter 'home level' data in columns A - G in all resident rows - values will be as for the first resident observed in that session. If doing another observation session immediately after the first, remember to enter all identifying data for the new session in columns A - G for the first resident observed in the new session. It will then be possible to go back later and enter the A - G data for the first session's residents

Some notes on coding

BEDSOCC

Information can be obtained from staff before or after observation. Aim to get a figure for the number of residents who would be counted for a fire alarm roll-call. This means excluding people who are away as temporary hospital in-patients or on holiday. Include day care attenders for observation sessions while they are in the home, i.e. ask number of attenders and approximate time of arrival and departure (of the day care group - do not attempt to track individual actual arrival/departure times). For example if doing observation sessions starting at 10, 11, 12 and 1 it is likely that day care attenders will be counted in the BEDSOCC total for 11, 12 and 1, but not for the 10 am session if they have not arrived by then. Ignore the complication of residents who come and go for short periods during the day - count them as present. The necessary arithmetic can be done and BEDSOCC totals entered at the end of the day's observation work.

ACTIVITY categories generally

All activity categories are designed to be mutually exclusive. Use 'awake' or 'sleeping/dozing' only when nothing else is going on. For example, if resident is asleep while being transported in a wheelchair code 'locomotion'. If the resident's behaviour changes in response to the appearance of an observer (e.g. he speaks to you) try to record the resident's activity/speech etc in relation to the split second before he became aware of your presence.

sleeping / dozing - awake

On occasion it may be difficult to decide between these options. Code according to whether or not the resident's eyes appear to be open. 'Awake' can apply to people standing as well as sitting.

performing self care activities

For example brushing hair/applying make-up.

listening to radio/ watching TV

Use this code where it appears that the resident is taking note of watching TV radio/TV - not where, e.g. TV is on in the background and being ignored. In cases of genuine doubt record the listening / watching code

<u>independent pursuit</u>

Use this code where resident is, e.g., reading, knitting, sewing or engaged in other solitary activity of recreational nature.

<u>chores</u>

Use this code for washing up, clearing dishes, mowing lawn etc - work about the house.

<u>group activity</u>

Use this code for all forms of social or recreational activity involving more than one *resident/visitor or member of staff* - e.g. card games, bingo, exercises, formal group discussion of any kind locomotion. This includes walking, wheeling, transferring which appears to be purposeful. Sometimes whether the movement has purpose will be unclear. If in doubt use this code.

<u>undirected activity</u>

Use this code for pacing etc. which appears to have no purpose. Give benefit of the doubt - only use this code if fairly sure that resident has no clear direction. Also use this for repetitive banging, clothes picking etc.

<u>eating / drinking</u>

Use this for any stage in a formal meal, e.g. resident sitting at dining table or individual trolley table set with cutlery, waiting to be served. If tea / coffee time use this code only for specific activity of being served or drinking tea / eating biscuits - not for mere presence in lounge while tea trolley being wheeled around.

<u>quiet speech</u>

All quiet one-way speech by the resident - includes talking to self, pets etc.

<u>loud speech</u>

All loud one-way speech by the resident. This includes calling for help, shouting - in some circumstances this may include arguments, i.e. if the resident is really shouting at somebody so not well described as conversation.

<u>being spoken to</u>

Resident is being spoken to by someone else and not responding.

<u>noise</u>

Screaming; repetitive calling ("Oh my God, Oh my God..." "Elsie.....Elsie.....Elsie...."). Differentiated from 'speaking loudly' because, if speech, does not appear coherent.

<u>conversation</u>

This includes all forms of apparently meaningful and directed 'verbal activity' where somebody appears to be listening and participating, Use this code if it is clear that conversation is taking place, even if resident is listening rather than speaking at moment of observation.

<u>other / uncodable</u>

For both activity and verbal categories it is possible to code 'other'. In these cases, where possible type a brief note in the Comments' column M.

<u>STAFF1 and STAFF2</u>

These are designed to record physical and/or verbal contact with one or two members of staff. 'Visiting professional' includes GP, chiropodist, Physiotherapist, district nurse, priest / minister. Some examples will elucidate this as well as illustrating use of the codes described above:

a) If the observed resident is being helped to walk by one nurse and one nursing assistant code

> ACTIVITY- 8 (locomotion)
> STAFF1 - 1 (nurse)
> STAFF2 - 2 (nursing assistant)

(b) If the resident is talking with one member of the domestic staff code

> ACTIVITY - 2 (awake)
> VERBAL - 5 (conversation)
> STAFF1 - 3 ('other' staff)
> STAFF2 - 0

(c) If the resident is knitting and not in verbal or physical contact of any kind code

> ACTIVITY - 5 (independent pursuit)
> VERBAL - 0
> STAFF1 - 0
> STAFF2 - 0

(d) If the resident is being helped to walk or exercise by a physiotherapist who is believed to be visiting, and no vocalisation of any kind is heard code

> ACTIVITY - 8 (locomotion)
> VERBAL - 0

STAFF1 - 4 (visiting professional)

STAFF2 - 0.

On the few occasions where this will arise it may be necessary to check (perhaps after the session) whether the professional was 'in house' or visiting.

(e) If the resident is pacing around the dining room repeatedly calling 'Oh my God help me'.. code

ACTIVITY - 8 (undirected activity)

VERBAL - 4 (noise)

STAFF1 - 0

STAFF2 - 0

(f) If the resident is in the lounge, rummaging in handbag, muttering quietly to self code

LOCATION - 2 (lounge)

ACTIVITY - 10 (other) (we cannot assume the rummaging is undirected or self care related)

VERBAL - 1   (quiet speech)

STAFF1 - 0

STAFF2 - 0

COMMENTS COLUMN M - handbag rummaging

Other equipment

On all observation sessions take an acetated coding card as well as the Psion, to act as a coding reminder; A spare set of batteries and a supply of coding sheets to be used with clipboard if necessary (i.e. in emergency due to Psion breakdown). Enter in the appropriate cell the name of the Psion file on which observation data for the particular session is recorded. Give this regularly to the Project Secretary for updating of the Observation Database.

Creating and naming data files; downloading data to desk - top computer

As soon as the database variable headings and the variable A - G identifying data have been entered, save as a file which will contain all the data for that day's observation. It is important to download and back up regularly so that data is not lost. Files should be named using the observer's initials and numbered in sequence. Files should be downloaded to desktop computer as frequently as possible to avoid loss of data. The Project Secretary will back up the data weekly on to disk.

To download plug Psion into black lead to desktop computer. Switch Psion on - display 'system' but do not open the relevant file. On computer open Psion Manager. Go to 'Internal'; then 'spr' and the files on the Psion spreadsheet should be revealed. Highlight the one to be copied; click on 'file' then 'copy and convert'. When the 'copy and convert' dialogue box appears check file is being saved as an Excel 5.0 file with suffix '.xls', also that it is going to c:\@psion\obsdata. If all well click 'ok' and confirm.

Appendix 2: Casemix Data Collection Sheet

Reproduced from the document used in the study (the page has been reduced in size for this volume).

"Case mix" data collection sheet

These are questions about the disabilities and care needs of all your residents. Please supply this information about all residents in the home, putting a number in each box alongside the initials of each resident (we do not need names - the initials are just for you to "keep track"). On continuation sheets please just insert "Resident Number" as a continuous sequence. Please first write your name and job title here _____

Today's date here _____ and the name of the Home here _____

Please "code" these items 1-4; 1 = "on own without difficulty". 2 = "on own with difficulty". 3 = "only with help". 4 = "not done"

Please "code" these items 1-3; 1 = Yes 2 = No 3 = sometimes

Res. Inits	Res No	do steps/ stairs	walk down road	walk indoors	transfer bed/ chair	go to WC	use WC	wash face & hands	bath, shower wash all over	dress/ undress	feed self	incont-inent?	short term memory problems?	disorien-tated, time,place person?	problem behaviour? (wandering, screaming, abusive?)
	1														
	2														
	3														
	4														
	5														
	6														
	7														
	8														
Cols	13-14	15	16	17	18	19	20	21	22	23	24	25	26	27	28

Appendix 3: Consent Procedures

Reproduced from the document used in the study (the page has been reduced in size for this volume).

The Quality of Life Study
Consent Procedures

1.When a new resident is admitted (or about to be admitted) to a participating home, the manager or a senior member of the home staff will tell the resident and any relatives involved that the home is taking part in the study; that the home will be giving the research team details of their name and admission date, and the relative's address, and that a researcher will be approaching them to ask them if they will agree to be included. At this time the member of home staff will give the resident and relative(s) copies of 'Project information for residents and relatives' and will point out that there is a telephone number if they wish to make further enquiries of the project team.

2. As soon as the team is notified of the new admission a letter will be sent to the resident's GP asking him or her to telephone within three working days in the event of wishing to exclude the resident on medical grounds. A member of the research team will speak to GPs or relatives who telephone and answer any queries.

3. After three working days a researcher will visit the newly admitted resident and will explain the study, referring to the project information which the resident has already received. One of three situations will prevail:-

(i) It is quite clear to the researcher that the resident is able to understand the explanation and able to give informed consent to take part in the study.

(ii) There is some doubt as to whether the explanation is understood (this may arise in cases of possible slight cognitive impairment or where there is sensory impairment which makes communication difficult).

(iii) It is clear to the researcher and to the home staff that the resident is unable to understand the explanation or give informed consent.

In situation (i) the researcher will give the resident a consent form for signature, ensuring that he or she also has a copy of the consent with project information on the reverse, to keep for future reference.

In situation (ii) the researcher will ask the manager or a member of staff to be present, or make whatever arrangements are necessary (e.g. signing interpreter etc) in order to ensure that the giving of informed consent is possible. If it is then deemed possible the resident will be asked to sign the consent, witnessed by the member of staff.

In situation (iii) the researcher and staff member will both sign an endorsement on the consent form to the effect that the resident was unable to understand the explanation of the study or to give informed consent, and showed no sign of dissent when asked to participate.

IN ALL CASES Interviewing will be terminated if the resident expresses a desire to withdraw or, in the case of cognitively impaired residents, if there are signs of distress indicating a desire to stop. No pressure will be put on anyone to take part; if in doubt researchers will not proceed.

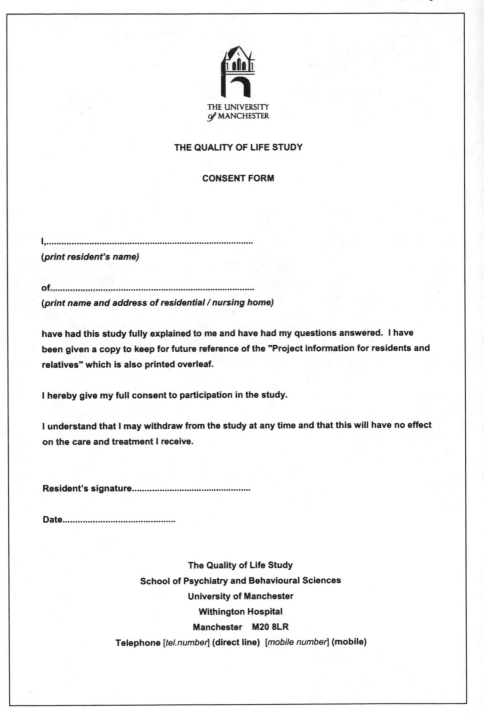

THE UNIVERSITY
of MANCHESTER

THE QUALITY OF LIFE STUDY

CONSENT FORM

I,..

(print resident's name)

of..

(print name and address of residential / nursing home)

have had this study fully explained to me and have had my questions answered. I have
been given a copy to keep for future reference of the "Project information for residents and
relatives" which is also printed overleaf.

I hereby give my full consent to participation in the study.

I understand that I may withdraw from the study at any time and that this will have no effect
on the care and treatment I receive.

Resident's signature...

Date...

The Quality of Life Study
School of Psychiatry and Behavioural Sciences
University of Manchester
Withington Hospital
Manchester   M20 8LR
Telephone [*tel.number*] (direct line) [*mobile number*] (mobile)

Appendix 4: Variables used in the Longitudinal Analysis

The following variables were chosen to be included in various parts of the longitudinal analysis. For ease of reference they are listed below, grouped into individual and home level variables. The subject matter, origin and measurement level of each variable is also given.

Individual level variables

Variable	Subject	Origin of data	Level of measure-ment
Age of resident	home records	ratio	
Social class	resident interview	nominal	
Sex	nominal		
Survival to follow up	home records	binary	
Survival time	home records	ratio	
MMSE score	cognitive impairment	resident interview	interval
MMSE category	cognitive impairment severity 'bands'	resident interview	ordinal
GDS-12R score	depression	resident interview	interval
GDS-12R 'caseness' threshold	depression	resident interview	binary
Barthel ADL score	dependency	informant interview	interval

Variable	Subject	Origin of data	Level of measure-ment
Barthel ADL category	dependency severity bands	informant interview	ordinal
Living situation satisfaction subscale	quality of life domain	resident interview	interval
Health satisfaction subscale	quality of life domain	resident interview	interval
Cantril's Ladder	quality of life global measure	resident interview analogue scale	interval
Spitzer Uniscale	quality of life global measure	interviewer assessed analogue scale	interval
Satisfaction with the prospect of living here a long time	quality of life single item	resident interview	binary
Satisfaction with opportunities for keeping occupied in the home	quality of life single item	resident interview	binary
Receipt of antidepressant medication (therapeutic dose)	home records	binary	
Satisfaction with pleasure from things done in the home	quality of life single item	resident interview	binary

Home level variables

Variable	Subject	Origin of data	Level of measure-ment
Home ownership sector		home questionnaire	nominal
Home type (nursing/ residential)		home questionnaire	nominal
'all carer' hours per occupied bed per day		home questionnaire	ratio
Maximum weekly charge for care		home questionnaire	ratio

Variable	Subject	Origin of data	Level of measurement
% residents who need help to use W.C.		home questionnaire	ratio
% disoriented residents		home questionnaire	ratio
% residents with behaviour problems		home questionnaire	ratio
% residents in private space		observation data	ratio
% inactive residents		observation data	ratio
Researcher home quality rating		researcher assessment	ordinal
'mean for home' SCES conflict sub-scale	social climate	staff questionnaire	interval
'mean for home' SCES cohesion sub-scale	social climate	staff questionnaire	interval
'mean for home' SCES resident influence' sub-scale	social climate	staff questionnaire	interval
'mean for home' SCES independence sub-scale	social climate	staff questionnaire	interval
'mean for home' SCES physical comfort sub-scale	social climate	staff questionnaire	interval
'mean for home' SCES organization sub-scale	social climate	staff questionnaire	interval
'mean for home' SCES self-disclosure sub-scale	social climate	staff questionnaire	interval
SCES cluster analysis groups	home quality category	nominal	
Staff sickness rate	home questionnaire	ratio	
Staff job satisfaction	staff questionnaire	interval	
Organisational stability	manager or owner change	manager interview	binary

Appendix 5: Abbreviations

For research instruments the first named author is given — see the bibliography and reference list.

ABS	Affect Balance Scale	Bradburn
ADL	Activities of Daily Living	
AMTS	Abbreviated Mental Test Score	Hodkinson
Barthel	Barthel Activities of Daily Living Index	Mahoney
BAS	Brief Assessment Schedule (see GMSS)	
CPA	Centre for Policy on Ageing	
Crichton Royal	Crichton Royal Behaviour Rating Scale	Wilkin
DCM	Dementia Care Mapping	
DSMIIIR	Diagnostic and Statistical Manual 3rd edition, revised	
GDS	Geriatric Depression Scale	Yesavage
GDS-12R	12 item GDS developed for this study	Sutcliffe
GDS-15	15 item Geriatric Depression Scale (see GDS)	
GHQ	General Health Questionnaire	Goldberg
GHQ-12	12 item General Health Questionnaire (see GHQ)	
GMSS	Geriatric Mental State Schedule	Copeland
GP	general (medical) practitioner	
GSCC	General Social Care Council	
HONOS-65+	Health of the Nation Outcome Scale (65+ version)	Curtis

ICD10	International Classification of Diseases	
LQOLP	Lancashire Quality of Life Profile	Oliver
LQOLP-R	LQOLP version developed for this study	
LSS	Life Satisfaction Scale	
MDS/RAI	Minimum data Set / Resident Assessment Instrument	Morris
MEAP	Multiphasic Environmental Assessment Procedure	Moos
MMSE	Mini Mental State Examination	Folstein
NSFOP	National Service Framework for Older People	
NVQ	National Vocational Qualification	
OBRA	Omnibus Budget Reconciliation Act	
QALY	Quality Adjusted Life Years	
SAP	Single Assessment Process	
RCN	Royal College of Nursing	
SCES	Sheltered Care Environment Scale	Moos
SCIE	Social Care Institute of Excellence	
TOPSS	National Training Organisation for Personal Social Services	

References and Bibliography

Abrams, M.A. (1973) Subjective social indicators, *Social Trends No.4*, Central Statistical Office, HMSO, London.

Ahmed, A.E., Nicholson, K.G. and Nguyen Van Tam, J.S. (1995) Reduction in mortality associated with influenza vaccine during 1989–1990 epidemic, *The Lancet*, 346, 8975, 591–595.

Albert, S.M. (1998) Progress in assessing health-related quality of life in people with Alzheimer's Disease, *The Quality of Life Newsletter*, 20, 13–16.

Albert, S.M., Del Castilo-Castaneda, C. and Sano, M. (1996) Quality of life in patients with Alzheimer's Disease as reported by patient proxies, *Journal of the American Geriatrics Society*, 44, 1342–1347.

Allen, I., Hogg, D. and Peace, S. (1992) *Elderly People: Choice, Participation and Satisfaction*, Policy Studies Institute, London.

Ames, D. (1990) Depression among elderly residents of local-authority residential homes — its nature and the efficacy of intervention, *British Journal of Psychiatry*, 156, 667–675.

Ames, D. (1994) Depression in nursing and residential homes, in Chiu, E. and Ames, D. (eds) *Functional Psychiatric Disorders of the Elderly*, Cambridge University Press, Cambridge.

Ames, D., Ashby, D., Mann, A.H. and Graham, N. (1988) Psychiatric illness in elderly residents of Part III homes in one London borough: prognosis and review, *Age and Ageing*, 17, 249–256.

Andrews, F.M. and McKennel, A.C. (1980) Measures of self-reported well-being; their affective, cognitive and other components, *Social Indicators Research*, 18, 127–155.

Andrews, F.M. and Withey, S.B. (1976) *Social Indicators of Well-being: Americans' Perceptions of Life Quality*, Plenum Press, New York.

Applegate, W.B., Miller, S.T., Graney, M.J., Elam, J.T., Burns, R. and Akins, D.E. (1990) A randomised, controlled trial of a geriatric assessment unit in a community rehabilitation hospital, *New England Journal of Medicine*, 322, 22, 1572–1578.

Audit Commission (2000a) *Forget Me Not: Mental Health Services for Older People*, Audit Commission, London.

Audit Commission (2000b) *The Way To Go Home: Rehabilitation and Remedial Services for Older People*, Audit Commission, London.

Audit Commission (2002) *Forget Me Not 2002: Developing Mental Health Services for Older People in England*, Audit Commission, London.

Bagley, H., Cordingley, L., Burns, A., Mozley, C.G., Sutcliffe, C., Challis, D. and Huxley, P. (2000) Recognition of depression in long term care facilities for older people: a comparison of qualified nurses and other care staff, *Journal of Clinical Nursing*, 9, 445–450.

Bagley, H., Challis, D., Hughes, J., Bhaduri, R., Burns, A., Reilly, S. and Wilson, K. (2002) Dementia care — the training needs of care staff in North West England, Discussion Paper M047, Personal Social Services Research Unit, University of Manchester and University of Kent at Canterbury.

Baldwin, R. (1997) Depressive illness, in Jacoby, R. and Oppenheimer, C. (eds) *Psychiatry in the Elderly*, Oxford University Press, Oxford.

Ball, M.M., Whittington, F.J., Perkins, M.M., Patterson, V.L., Hollingsworth, C., King, S.V. and Combs, B.L. (2000) Quality of life in assisted living facilities: viewpoints of residents, *Journal of Applied Gerontology*, 19, 3, 304–325.

Ballard, C., O'Brien, J., James, I., Mynt, P., Lana, M., Potkins, D., Reichelt, K., Lee, L., Swann, A. and Fossey, J. (2001a) Quality of life for people with dementia living in residential and nursing home care: the impact of performance on activities of daily living, behavioural and psychological symptoms, language skills and psychotropic drugs, *International Psychogeriatrics*, 13, 1, 93–106.

Ballard, C., Fossey, J., Chithramohan, R.H., Burns, A., Thompson, P., Tadros, G. and Fairbairn, A. (2001b) Quality of care in private sector and NHS facilities for people with dementia: cross sectional survey, *British Medical Journal*, 323, 426–427.

Balogh, R., Bond, S., Simpson, A. and Quinn, H. (1993) *An Analysis of Instruments and Tools Used in Psychiatric Nursing Audit*, Centre for Health Services Research, University of Newcastle.

Barba, B.E., Tesh, A.S. and Courts, N.F. (2002) Promoting thriving in nursing homes, *Journal of Gerontological Nursing*, 28, 3, 7–13.

Barry, M.M., Crosby, C. and Bogg, J. (1993) Methodological issues in evaluating the quality of life of long stay psychiatric patients, *Journal of Mental Health*, 2, 43–56.

Bass, B.M. (1985) *Leadership and Performance Beyond Expectations*, Free Press, New York.

Bebbington, P., Brown, P., Darton, R. and Netten, A (1996) Survey of Admissions to Residential Care: the lifetime risk of entering residential or nursing home care for elderly people, Discussion Paper 1230/2, Personal Social Services Research Unit, University of Kent at Canterbury.

Bell, M. and Goss, A.J. (2001) Recognition, assessment and treatment of depression in geriatric nursing home residents, *Clinical Excellence for Nurse Practitioners*, 5, 1, 26–36.

Benjamin, L. and Spector, J. (1990) The relationships of staff, resident and environmental characteristics to stress experienced by staff caring for the dementing, *International Journal of Geriatric Psychiatry*, 5, 25–31.

Bergner, M., Bobbitt, R.A., Kressel, S., Pollard, W.E., Gilson, B.S. and Morris, J.R. (1976) The Sickness Impact Profile: conceptual formulation and methodology for the development of a health status measure, *International Journal of Health Services*, 6, 3, 393–415.

Bhaduri, R. (ed.) (2001) *Caring with Confidence: A Handbook for Training in Dementia Care for Nursing and Care Assistants in Continuing Care Homes*, Personal Social Services Research Unit, University of Manchester.

Black, D. and Bowman, C. (1997) Community institutional care for frail elderly people — time to restructure professional responsibility, *British Medical Journal*, 315, 441–442.

Blanchard, M., Waterreus, A. and Mann, A.H. (1995) The effect of primary care nurse intervention upon older people screened as depressed, *International Journal of Geriatric Psychiatry*, 10, 289–298.

Bland, R., Bland, R., Cheetham, J., Lapsley, I. and Llewellyn, S. (1992) *Residential Homes for Elderly People: Their Costs and Quality*, HMSO, Edinburgh.

Blessed, G., Tomlinson, B. and Roth, M. (1968) The association between quantitative measures of dementia and senile change in the grey matter of elderly subjects, *British Journal of Psychiatry*, 114, 797–811.

Bond, J., Bond, S., Donaldson, C., Gregson, B. and Atkinson, A. (1989) Evaluation of an innovation in the continuing care of very frail elderly people, *Ageing and Society*, 9, 347–381.

Booth, T. (1985) *Home Truths: Old People's Homes and the Outcome of Care*, Gower, Aldershot.

Borrill, C.S., Wall, T.D., West, M.A., Hardy, G.E., Shapiro, D.A., Carter, A., Golya, D.A. and Haynes, C.E. (1996) *Mental Health of the Workforce in NHS Trusts. Phase 1 Final Report*, Institute of Work Psychology, University of Sheffield/ Department of Psychology, University of Leeds.

Bowers, J., Jorm, A.F., Henderson, S. and Harris, P. (1990) General practitioners' detection of depression and dementia in elderly patients, *The Medical Journal of Australia*, 153, 192–196.

Bowling A. (1995) What things are important in people's lives? A survey of the public's judgements to inform scales of health related quality of life, *Social Science and Medicine*, 41, 1447–1462.

Bowling, A. (1997) *Measuring Health: A Review of Quality of Life Measurement Scales*, Buckingham, Open University Press.

Bowling, A. (1998) Measuring health related quality of life among older people. Editorial, *Aging and Mental Health*, 2, 1, 5–6.

Bowling A. and Formby, J. (1992) Hospital and nursing home care for the elderly in an inner city health district, *Nursing Times*, 88, 13, 51–54.

Bowling, A. and Windsor, J. (2001) Towards the good life: a population survey of dimensions of quality of life, *Journal of Happiness Studies*, 2, 55–81.

Bowling, A., Formby, J. and Grant, K. (1992) Accidents in elderly care: a randomised controlled trial (Part 3), *Nursing Standard*, 6, 31, 25–27.

Bowns, I., Challis, D. and Tong, M.S. (1991) Case finding in elderly people: validation of a postal questionnaire, *British Journal of General Practice*, 41, 100–104.

Bradburn, N.M. (1969) *The Structure of Psychological Well-being*, Aldine Publishing, Chicago.

Braekhaus, A., Laake, K. and Engedal K. (1992) The Mini-Mental State Examination: identifying the most efficient variables for detecting cognitive impairment in the elderly, *The American Geriatrics Society*, 40, 1139–1145.

Breuer, B., Wallenstein, S., Feinberg, C., Camargo, M.J. and Libow, L.S. (1998) Assessing life expectancies of older nursing home residents, *Journal of the American Geriatrics Society*, 46, 8, 954–961.

Brocklehurst, J., Carty, M. and Leeming, J. (1978) Care of the elderly: medical screening of old people accepted for residential care, *The Lancet*, ii, 141–142.

Brooke, V. (1989) How elders adjust, *Geriatric Nursing*, 10, 2, 66–68.

Bruce, E., Surr, C. and Tibbs, M. (2002) *A Special Kind of Care: Improving Well-Being in People Living With Dementia. A Report by MHA Care Group and the Bradford Dementia Group*, MHA Care Group, Derby.

Buchanan, A.E. and Brock, D.W. (1989) *Deciding for Others: The Ethics of Surrogate Decision Making*, Cambridge University Press, Cambridge.

Burke, W.J., Nichter, R.L., Roccaforte, W.H. and Wengel, S.P. (1992) A prospective evaluation of the Geriatric Depression Scale in an outpatient geriatric assessment center, *Journal of the American Geriatrics Society*, 40, 1227–1230.

Burns, A. and Lewis, G. (1993) Survival in dementia, in Burns, A. (ed.) *Ageing in Dementia: A Methodological Review*, Edward Arnold, London.

Burns, A., Jacobi, R. and Luther, B. (1990) Cause of death in Alzheimer's disease, *Age and Ageing*, 19, 341–344.

Burns, A., Beevor, A., Lelliot, P., Wing, J., Blakey, A., Orrell, M., Mullinga, J. and Hadden, S. (1999) Health of the Nation Outcome Scales for elderly people (HoNOS 65+), *British Journal of Psychiatry*, 174, 435–438.

Bury, M. and Holme, A. (1990) Researching very old people, in Peace, S.M. (ed.) (1990) *Researching Social Gerontology: Concepts, Methods and Issues*, Sage, London.

Campbell, A., Converse, P.E. and Rogers, W.L. (1976) *The Quality of American Life*, Russell Sage, New York.

Campbell, A. (1981) *The Sense of Well-being in America*, McGraw-Hill, New York.

Campbell Stern, M., Jagger, C., Clarke, M., Anderson, J., McGrother, C., Battock, T. and McDonald, C. (1993) Residential care for elderly people: a decade of change, *British Medical Journal*, 306, 6881, 827–830.

Cantril, H. (1965) *The Pattern of Human Concerns*, Rutgers University Press, New Brunswick, New Jersey.

Caplan, R.D. (1971) *Organizational Stress and Individual Strain: A Social Psychological Study of Risk Factors in Coronary Heart Disease Among Administrators, Engineers and Scientists*, Institute of Social Research, University Microfilms 72–14822, University of Michigan, Ann Arbor, Michigan.

Care Standards Act (2000) (2000 c.14) HMSO, London.

Cartwright, A. (1964) *Human Relations and Hospital Care*, Routledge and Kegan Paul, London.

Cartwright, A. (1978) Professionals as responders: variations in and effects of response rates to questionnaires 1961–1977, *British Medical Journal*, ii, 1419–1421.

Centre for Policy on Ageing (1984) *Home Life: A Code of Practice for Residential Care*, Centre for Policy on Ageing, London.

Challiner, Y., Watson, R., Julious, S. and Philip, I. (1994) A postal survey of the quality of long term institutional care, *International Journal of Geriatric Psychiatry*, 9, 619–625.

Challis, D. (1981) Measurement of outcome in social care of the elderly, *Journal of Social Policy*, 10, 2, 179–208.

Challis, D. and Darton, R. (1990) Evaluation research in social gerontology, in Peace, S. (ed.) *Researching Social Gerontology*, Sage, London.

Challis, D. and Davies, B. (1986) *Case Management in Community Care*, Gower, Aldershot.

Challis, D. and Hughes, J. (2002) Frail old people at the margins of care: some recent research findings, *British Journal of Psychiatry*, 180, 126–130.

Challis, D., Knapp, M. and Davies, B.P. (1988) Cost effectiveness evaluation in social care, in Lishman, J. (ed.) *Evaluation*, Jessica Kingsley, London.

Challis, D., Darton, R., Johnson, L., Stone, M. and Traske, K. (1995) *Care management and health care of older people*, Ashgate, Aldershot.

Challis, D., Carpenter, I. and Traske, K. (1996) *Assessment in Continuing Care Homes: Towards a National Standard Instrument*, PSSRU/Joseph Rowntree Foundation, University of Kent at Canterbury.

Challis, D., von Abendorff, R., Brown, P. and Chesterman, J. (1997) Care management and dementia: an evaluation of the Lewisham Intensive Case Management Scheme, in Hunter, S (ed.) *Dementia Challenges and New Directions*, Jessica Kingsley, London.

Challis, D., Darton, R. and Stewart, K. (1998) Linking community care and health care: a new role for secondary health care services, in Challis, D., Darton, R. and Stewart, K. (eds) *Community Care, Secondary Health Care and Care Management*, Ashgate, Aldershot.

Challis, D., Stewart, K., Sturdy, D. and Worden, A. (eds) (2000a) *UK Long Term Care Resident Assessment User's Manual, MDS/RAI UK*, InterRAI UK, York.

Challis, D., Mozley, C.G., Sutcliffe, C., Bagley, H., Price, L., Burns, A., Huxley, P. and Cordingley, L. (2000b) Dependency in older people recently admitted to care homes, *Age and Ageing*, 29, 255–260.

Challis, D., Chesterman, J., Luckett, R., Stewart, K. and Chessum, R. (2002a) *Care Management in Social and Primary Health Care: The Gateshead Community Care Scheme*, Ashgate, Aldershot.

Challis, D., Reilly, S., Hughes, J., Burns, A., Gilchrist, H. and Wilson, K. (2002b) Policy, organisation and practice of specialist old age psychiatry in England, *International Journal of Geriatric Psychiatry*, 17, 1018–1026.

Chambers, L.W. (1984) A self-monitoring method of resident care quality assurance in long-term care facilities, *Canadian Journal on Ageing*, 2, 3, 137–151.

Chambers, L.W. (1986) *Quality Assurance in Long Term Care: Policy, Research and Measurement*, International Center of Social Gerontology on behalf of the World Health Organisation, Paris.

Charlesworth, A. and Wilkin, D. (1982) Dependency among old people in geriatric wards, psychogeriatric wards and residential homes 1977–1981, Research Report No. 6, Department of Psychiatry and Community Medicine, University of Manchester.

Chenitz, W.C. (1983) Entry into a nursing home as status passage: a theory to guide nursing practice, *Geriatric Nursing*, 4, 2, 92–97.

Clark, P. and Bowling, A. (1989) Observational study of quality of life in NHS nursing homes and a long-stay ward for the elderly, *Ageing and Society*, 9, 123–148.

Clark, P. and Bowling, A. (1990) Quality of everyday life in long stay institutions for the elderly. An observational study of long stay hospital and nursing home care, *Social Science and Medicine*, 30, 11, 1201–1210.

Clark, P.G. (1995) Quality of life, values and team work in geriatric care, *The Gerontologist*, 35, 3, 402–411.

Cm 4014 (1998) *Modern Local Government: In Touch with the People*, The Stationery Office, London.

Cm 4169 (1998) *Modernising Social Services*, The Stationery Office, London.

Cm 4818–1, (2000) *The NHS Plan. The Government's Response to the Royal Commission on Long Term Care*, The Stationery Office, London.

Coast, J., Peters, T.J., Richards, S.H. and Gunnell, D.J. (1998) Use of the EuroQol among elderly acute care patients, *Quality of Life Research*, 7, 1–10.

Cohen-Mansfield, J. and Werner, P. (1999) Outdoor wandering parks for persons with dementia: a survey of characteristics and use, *Alzheimer Disease and Associated Disorders*, 13, 2, 109–117.

Cohen-Mansfield, J., Marx, M.S., Lipson, S. and Werner, P. (1999) Predictors of mortality in nursing home residents, *Journal of Clinical Epidemiology*, 52, 4, 273–280.

Collin, C., Wade D.T., Davies S. and Horne V. (1988) The Barthel ADL Index: a reliability study, *International Disability Studies*, 10, 61–63.

Cook, J.D. and Wall, T.D. (1980) New work attitude measures of trust, organisational commitment and personal need non-fulfilment, *Journal of Occupational Psychology*, 53, 147–153.

Copeland, J.R.M., Kelleher, M.J., Kellett, J.M., Gourlay, A.J., Gurland, B.J., Fleiss, J.L. and Sharpe, L. (1976) A semi-structured clinical interview for the assessment of diagnosis and mental state in the elderly. The Geriatric Mental State Schedule: I. Development and reliability, *Psychological Medicine*, 6, 439–449.

Copeland, J.R.M., Dewey, M.E. and Griffiths-Jones, H.M. (1986) A computerized psychiatric diagnostic system and case nomenclature for elderly subjects: GMS and AGECAT, *Psychological Medicine*, 16, 89–99.

Copeland, J.R., Dewey, M.E., Henderson, A.S., Kay, D.W., Neal, C.D., Harrison, M.A., William, C., Forshaw, D. and Shiwach, R. (1988) The Geriatric Mental State (GMS) used in the community: replication studies of the computerised diagnosis AGECAT, *Psychological Medicine*, 18, 10, 219–223.

Corbett, J. (1997) Provision of prescribing advice for nursing and residential home patients, *Pharmaceutical Journal*, 259, 6960, 422–424.

Cox, C.L., Kaeser, L., Montgomery, A.C. and Marion, L. (1991) Quality of life nursing care: an experimental trial in long-term care, *Journal of Gerontological Nursing*, 17, 4, 6–11.

Cox, D.R. and Oaks, D. (1984) *Analysis of Survival Data*, Chapman and Hall, London.

Cuipers, P. (2001) Mortality and depressive symptoms in inhabitants of residential homes, *International Journal of Geriatric Psychiatry*, 16, 131–138.

Cumming, E. and Henry, W. (1961) *Growing Old*, Basic Books, New York.

Curtis, R. and Beevor, A. (1995) Health of the Nation Outcome Scales, in Wing J.K. (ed.) *Measurement for Mental Health: Contributions from the College Research Unit*, Royal College of Psychiatrists, London.

Darton, R.A. and Brown, P. (1997) Survey of Admissions to Residential Care Analyses of Six Month Follow-up, Discussion Paper 1340, Personal Social Services Research Unit, University of Kent at Canterbury.

D'Ath, P., Katona, P., Mullan, E., Evans, S. and Katona, C. (1994) Screening, detection and management of depression in elderly primary care attenders. I: The acceptability and performance of the 15 item Geriatric Depression Scale (GDS-15) and the development of shorter versions, *Family Practitioner*, 11, 3, 260–266.

Davies, B.P. and Knapp, M. (1980) *Old Peoples Homes and the Production of Welfare*, Routledge and Kegan Paul, London.

Davies, S. (2001) The care needs of older people and family caregivers in continuing care settings, in Nolan, M., Davies, S. and Grant, G. (eds) *Working with Older People and Their Families. Key Issues in Policy and Practice*, Open University Press, Buckingham.

Davies, S., Slack, R., Laker, S. and Philp, I. (1999) The educational preparation of staff in nursing homes: relationship with resident autonomy, *Journal of Advanced Nursing*, 29, 1, 208–217.

de Veer, A. and Kerkstra, A. (2001) Feeling at home in nursing homes, *Journal of Advanced Nursing*, 35, 3, 427–434.

Dean, R., Proudfoot, R. and Lindesay, J. (1993) The Quality of Interactions Schedule (QUIS): development, reliability and use in evaluation of two domus settings, *International Journal of Geriatric Psychiatry*, 8, 819–826.

Denham, M.J. (1991) Quality of life: assessment and improvement, in Denham, M. (ed.) *Care of the Long-Stay Elderly Patient (2nd edition)*, Chapman and Hall, London.

Department of Health (1992) *The Health of the Nation. A Strategy for Health in England*, HMSO, London.

Department of Health (1997) *Better Services for Vulnerable People*, EL(97)62, CI(97)24, HMSO, London.

Department of Health (1998a) *A First Class Service — Quality in the New NHS*, Department of Health, London.

Department of Health (1998b) *The Quality Protects Programme: Transforming Children's Services*, LAC(98) 28, Department of Health, London.

Department of Health (1999) *Fit for the Future? National Required Standards for Residential and Nursing Homes for Older People Consultation Document*, Department of Health, London.

Department of Health (2000) *A Quality Strategy for Social Care*, LASSL(2000)9, Department of Health, London.

Department of Health (2001a) *Care Homes for Older People: National Minimum Standards*, The Stationery Office, London.

Department of Health (2001b) *National Service Framework for Older People*, Department of Health, London.

Department of Health (2001c) *National Service Framework for Older People, Medicines and Older People; Implementing Medicines Related Aspects of the NSF for Older People*, Department of Health, London.

Department of Health (2001d) *Intermediate Care*, HSC 2001/01, LAC(2001)01, Department of Health, London.

Department of Health (2001e) *Community Care Statistics 2001*, Department of Health, London, *http://www.doh.gov.uk/public/sb0129.htm*.

Department of Health (2001f) *Guidance on Free Nursing Care in Nursing Homes*, HSC 2001/017, Department of Health, London.

Department of Health (2002a) *Guidance on the Single Assessment Process for Older People*, HSC 2002/001, LAC(2002)1, Department of Health, London.

Department of Health (2002b) *Care Homes for Older People and Younger Adults, National Minimum Standards for Care Homes for Older People — Proposed Amended Environmental Standards*, Department of Health, London.

Department of Health (2002c) *Single Assessment Process: Tools and Scales*, Department of Health, *http://www.doh.gov.uk/scg/sap/toolsandscales.index.htm*.

Department of Health /Social Services Inspectorate (1989) *Homes are For Living In*, HMSO, London.

Devis, T. and Rooney, C. (1997) The time taken to register a death, *Population Trends*, 88, Summer, 48–55.

Dewey, M.E., Davidson, I.A. and Copeland, J.R. (1993) Expressed wish to die and mortality in older people: a community replication, *Age and Ageing*, 22, 109–113.

Donabedian, A. (1980) *Explorations in Quality Assessment and Monitoring Volume I: The Definition of Quality and Approaches to its Assessment*, Health Administration Press, Ann Arbor.

Donaldson, C., Atkinson, A., Bond, J. and Wright, K. (1988) QALYs and long-term care for elderly people in the UK: scales for assessment of quality of life, *Age and Ageing*, 17, 379–387.

Downs, M. (1997) The emergence of the person in dementia research, *Ageing and Society*, 17, 597–607.

Draper, B., Brodaty, H., Low, L.F., Saab, D., Richards, V. and Paton, H. (2001) Use of psychotropics in Sydney nursing homes: associations with depression, psychosis and behavioural disturbances, *International Psychogeriatrics*, 13, 1, 107–120.

Draper, P. (1992) Quality of life as quality of being: an alternative to the subject-object dichotomy, *Journal of Advanced Nursing*, 17, 965–970.

Drew, J.C. and Brooke, V. (1999) Changing a legacy: The Eden Alternative Nursing Home, *Annals of Long-Term Care*, 7, 3, 115–121.

Eagles, J.M., Beattie, J.A.G., Restall, D.B., Rawlinson F., Hagen S. and Ashcroft, G.W. (1990) Relation between cognitive impairment and early death in the elderly, *British Medical Journal*, 300, 239–240.

Euroqol Group (1990) EuroQoL (c) — a new facility for the measurement of health-related quality of life, *Health Policy*, 16, 3, 199–208.

Evans, J.G. (1992) Quality of life assessments and elderly people, in Hopkins A. (ed.) *Measures of the Quality of Life*, Royal College of Physicians, Oxprint Ltd., Oxford.

Evans, G., Hughes, B., Wilkin, D. with Jolley, D. (1981) The management of mental and physical impairment in non-specialist homes for the elderly, Research Report No 4, Department of Psychiatry and Community Medicine, University of Manchester.

Fallowfield, L. (1991) *The Quality of Life: the Missing Measurement in Health Care*, Paul and Company, New York.

Farquhar, M. (1995a) Definitions of quality of life: a taxonomy, *Journal of Advanced Nursing*, 22, 502–508.

Farquhar, M. (1995b) Elderly people's definitions of quality of life, *Social Science and Medicine*, 41, 10, 1439–1446.

Flacker, J. and Kiely, D. (1998) Practical approach to identifying mortality-related factors in established long term care residents, *Journal of the American Geriatrics Society*, 46, 8, 1012–1015.

Fleishman, R., Mizrahi, G., Bar-Giora, M., Mandelson, J. and Yuz, F. (1995) *Surveillance of Institutions for the Semi-Independent and Frail Elderly*, JDC Brookdale Institute of Gerontology and Human Development/Ministry of Labor and Social Affairs Service for the Aged, Jerusalem.

Fletcher, A.E, Dickinson, E.J. and Philp, I. (1992) Quality of life instrument for everyday use with elderly patients, *Age and Ageing*, 21, 142–150.

Folstein, M.F., Folstein, S.E. and McHugh, P.R. (1975) Mini-Mental State: a practical method for grading the cognitive state of patients for the clinician, *Journal of Psychiatric Research*, 12, 189–198.

Franklin, J.L., Simmons, J., Solovitz, B., Clemons, J.R. and Miller, G.E. (1986) Assessing quality of life of the mentally ill. A three dimensional model, *Evaluation and the Health Professions*, 9, 3, 376–388.

Fried, T.R. and Mor, V. (1997) Frailty and hospitalisation of long term stay nursing home residents, *Journal of the American Geriatric Society*, 45, 3, 265–269.

Frischer, M. (1991) Trends in morbidity and general practitioner's workload for middle aged and elderly people from 1956 to 1982, *The Journal of Public Health Medicine*, 13, 3, 198–203.

Freedman, N., Bucci, W. and Elkowitz, E. (1982) Depression in a family practice elderly population, *Journal of American Geriatric Society*, 30, 6, 372–377.

Frytak, J. (2000) Assessment of quality of life, in Kane, R. and Kane, R. (eds) *Assessing Older Persons: Measures, Meaning and Practical Applications*, Oxford U.P, New York.

Furniss, L., Burns, A., Craig, S., Scobie, S., Cooke, J. and Faragher, B. (2000) Effects of a pharmacist's medication review in nursing homes, *British Journal of Psychiatry*, 176, 563–567.

Gallichon, M. (2002) A diabetes education initiative for residential care home staff, *Professional Nurse*, 17, 7, 432–435.

Gelder, M.G., Gath, D. and Mayou, R. (1989) *Oxford Textbook of Psychiatry*, 2nd Edition, Oxford University Press, Oxford.

Gentile, K.M. (1991) A review of the literature on interventions and quality of life in the frail elderly, in Birren, J.E., Lubben, J.E., Rowe, J.C. and Deutchman, D.E. (eds) *The Concept and Measurement of Quality of Life in the Frail Elderly*, Academic Press: San Diego.

George, L.K. and Bearon, L.B. (1980) *Quality of Life In Older Persons: Meaning and Measurement*. Human Sciences Press, New York.

Gerety, M.B., Williams, J.W., Mulrwo, C.D., Cornell, J.E., Kadri, A.A., Rosenberg, J., Chiodo, L.K. and Long, M. (1994) Performance of case-finding tools for depression in the nursing home: influence of clinical and functional characteristics and selection of optimal threshold scores, *Journal of the American Geriatrics Society*, 42, 1103–1109.

Geron, S.M. (1991) Regulating the behaviour of nursing homes through positive incentives: an analysis of Illinois' Quality Incentive Program (QUIP), *Gerontologist*, 31, 292–301.

Geron, S.M. (1998) Assessing the satisfaction of older adults with long-term care services: measurement and design challenges for social work, *Research on Social Work Practice*, 8, 1, 103–119.

Gibbs, I. and Sinclair, I. (1992a) Consistency: a pre-requisite for inspecting old people's homes, *British Journal of Social Work*, 22, 541–549.

Gibbs, I. and Sinclair, I. (1992b) Residential care for elderly people: the correlates of quality, *Ageing and Society*, 12, 4, 463–482.

Gilleard, C. (1992) Community care services for the elderly mentally infirm, in Jones, G.M.M. and Miesen, B.M.L. (eds) *Care-Giving in Dementia: Research and Applications*, Routledge, London.

Glendinning, C., Jacobs, S., Alborz, A. and Hann, M. (2002) A survey of access to medical services in nursing and residential homes in England, *British Journal of General Practice*, 52, 545–548.

Godlove, C., Dunn, G. and Wright, H. (1980) Caring for old people in New York and London: the 'Nurses' Aide' interviews, *Journal of the Royal Society of Medicine*, 73, 713–723.

Godlove, C., Richard, L. and Rodwell, G. (1982) *Time for Action: An Observation Study of Elderly People in Four Different Care Environments*, Joint Unit for Social Services Research, Sheffield University/Community Care.

Goldberg, D. and Huxley, P. (1992) *Common Mental Disorders: A Bio-Social Model*, Tavistock/Routledge, London.

Goldberg, D. and Williams, P. (1988) *A User's Guide to the General Health Questionnaire*, NFER-Nelson Publishing, Windsor.

Goldberg, E.M. and Connelly, N. (1982) *The Effectiveness of Social Care for the Elderly*, Heinemann, London.

Granger, C.V., Albrecht, G.L. and Byron, B.H. (1979) Outcome of comprehensive medical rehabilitation: measurement by PULSES profile and the Barthel Index, *Archives of Physical and Medical Rehabilitation*, 60, 145–153.

Grau, L., Chandler, B. and Saunders, C. (1995) Nursing home residents' perceptions of the quality of their care, *Journal of Psychosocial Nursing and Mental Health Services*, 33, 34–41.

Grundy, E. and Bowling, A. (1999) Enhancing the quality of extended life years. Identification of the oldest old with a very good and very poor quality of life, *Aging and Mental Health*, 3, 3, 199–212

Gurland, B., Cross, P., Defiguerido, J., Shannon, M., Mann, A.H., Jenkins, R., Bennett, R., Wilder, D., Wright, H., Killeffer, E., Godlove, C., Thompson, P., Ross, M. and Deming, W.E. (1979) A cross national comparison of the institutionalized elderly in the cities of New York and London, *Psychological Medicine*, 9, 781–788.

Gurvich, T. and Cunningham, J.A. (2000) Appropriate use of psychotropic drugs in nursing homes, *American Family Physician*, 61, 1437–1446.

Hackman, J.R. and Oldham, G.R. (1975) Development of the job diagnostics survey, *Journal of Applied Psychology*, 60, 159–170.

Hansebo, G., Kihlgren, M., Ljunggren, G. and Winblad, B. (1998) Staff views on the Resident Assessment Instrument, RAI/MDS, in nursing homes, and the use of the Cognitive Performance Scale, CPS, in different levels of care in Stockholm, Sweden, *Journal of Advanced Nursing*, 28, 3, 642–653.

Hawes, C., Morris, J.N., Phillips, C.D., Fries, B.E., Murphy, K. and Mor, V. (1997) Development of the Nursing Home Resident Assessment Instrument in the USA, *Age and Ageing*, 26-S2, 19–25.

Henderson, A.S. (1986) Epidemiology of mental illness, in *Mental Health in the Elderly: A Review of Present State of Research*, Springer, Berlin.

Henderson, S., Byrne, D.G. and Duncan-Jones, P. (1981) *Neurosis and the Social Environment*, Academic Press, Sydney.

Hertzberg, A. and Ekman, S. (2000) 'We, not them and us?' Views on the relationships and interactions between staff and relatives of older people permanently living in nursing homes, *Journal of Advanced Nursing*, 31, 3, 614–622.

Hertzberg, A., Ekman, S. and Axelsson, K. (2001) Staff activities and behaviour are the source of many feelings: relatives' interactions and relationships with staff in nursing homes, *Journal of Clinical Nursing*, 10, 3, 380–388.

Heston, L.L., Gerrard, J., Makris, L., Kane, R.L., Cooper, S., Dunham, T. and Zelterman, D. (1992) Inadequate treatment of depressed nursing home elderly, *Journal of the American Geriatric Society*, 40, 11, 1117–1122.

HMSO (1975) *Statistical Review of England and Wales, 1973*, London, HMSO.

Hodkinson, H.M. (1972) Evaluation of a mental test score for assessment of mental impairment in the elderly, *Age and Ageing*, 1, 233–238.

Hodkinson, H.M. (1973) Mental impairment in the elderly, *Journal of the Royal College of Physicians*, 7, 305–317.

Hooijer, C., Dinkgreve, M., Jonker, C., Lindebroom, J. and Kay, D. (1992a) Short screening tests for dementia in the elderly population I: A comparison between AMTS, MMSE, MSQ and SPMSQ, *International Journal of Geriatric Psychiatry*, 7, 559–571.

Hooijer, C., Dinkgreve, M., Jonker, C., Lindebroom, J. and Kay, D. (1992b) Short screening tests for dementia in the elderly population. II: The combined use of more than one test, *International Journal of Geriatric Psychiatry*, 7, 827–833.

Hopkins, A., Brocklehurst, J. and Dickinson, E. (1992) *The CARE Scheme (Continuous Assessment Review and Evaluation): Clinical Audit of Long-Term Care of Elderly People*, Royal College of Physicians of London, London.

Horgas A.L. and Tsai, P.F. (1998) Analgesic drug prescription and use in cognitively impaired nursing home residents, *Nursing Research*, 47, 4, 235–242.

Hughes, B. (1990) Quality of life, in Peace, S. (ed.) *Researching Social Gerontology*, Sage, London.

Hunt, S.M., McKenna, S.P., McEwan, J., Backett, E.M., Williams, J. and Papp, E. (1980) A quantitative approach to perceived health status: a validation study, *Journal of Epidemiology and Community Health*, 34, 4, 281–286.

Hunt, S.M., McEwan, J. and McKenna, S.P. (1986) *Measuring Health Status*, Croom Helm, London.

Huxley, P. (1998) Outcomes management in mental health: a brief review, *Journal of Mental Health*, 7, 3, 273–283.

Iliffe, S., Booroff, A., Gallivan, S., Goldenberg, E., Morgan, P. and Haines, A. (1990) Screening for cognitive impairment in the elderly using The Mini-Mental State Examination, *British Journal of General Practice*, 40, 336, 277–279.

Jackson, R. and Baldwin, B. (1993) Detecting depression in elderly medically ill patients: the use of the Geriatric Depression Scale compared with medical and nursing observations, *Age and Ageing*, 22, 349–353.

Jacobs, S. and Rummery, K. (2002) Nursing homes in England and their capacity to provide rehabilitation and intermediate care services, *Social Policy and Administration*, 36, 735–752.

Jacobs, S., Alborz, A., Glendinning, C. and Hann, M. (2001) *Health Services for Homes: A Survey of Access to NHS Services in Residential and Nursing Homes for Older People in England*, National Primary Care Research and Development Centre, University of Manchester.

Jacqmin-Gadda, H., Fabrigoule, C., Commenges, D. and Dartigues, J.F. (1997) A five year longitudinal study of the MMSE in normal aging, *American Journal of Epidemiology*, 145, 6, 498–506.

Johnson, M.L. (1972) Self perception of need amongst the elderly: an analysis of illness behaviour, *Sociological Review*, 20, 521- 531.

Kafonek, S., Ettinger, W.H., Roca, R., Kittner, S., Taylor, N. and German, P.S. (1989) Instruments for screening for depression and dementia in a long-term care facility, *Journal of the American Geriatrics Society*, 37, 29–34.

Kane, R.A. (2001) Long-term care and a good quality of life: bringing them closer together, *The Gerontologist*, 41, 3, 293–304.

Kane, R.A. and Kane, R.L. (1987) *Long Term Care. Principles, Programs, and Policies*, Springer, New York.

Kane, R.A. and Kane, R.L. (1988) Long-term care: variations on a quality assurance theme, *Inquiry*, Spring, 132–146.

Kane, R.A., Giles, K., Lawton, M.P. and Kane, R.L. (1999) *Development of Measures and Indicators of Quality of Life in Nursing Homes: Wave 1. Report to the Health Care Financing Administration*, University of Minnesota School of Public Health, Minneapolis.

Kane, R.L., Bell, R., Riegler, S., Wilson, A. and Keeler, E. (1983) Predicting the outcomes of nursing home patients, *The Gerontologist*, 23, 200–206.

Karon, S. and Zimmerman, D. (1996) Using indicators to structure quality improvement initiatives in long-term care, *Quality Management in Health Care*, 4, 3, 54–66.

Kayser-Jones, J.S. (1986) Open-ward accommodations in a long-term care facility; the elderly's point of view, *The Gerontologist*, 21, 1, 63–69.

Kerrison, H.K. and Pollock, A.M. (2001a) Absent voices compromise the effectiveness of nursing home regulation: a critique of regulatory reform in the UK nursing home industry, *Health and Social Care in the Community*, 9, 6, 490–494.

Kerrison, H.K. and Pollock, A.M. (2001b) Regulating nursing homes: caring for older people in the private sector, *British Medical Journal*, 323, 566–569.

Kitwood, T. and Bredin, K. (1994) *Evaluating dementia care the DCM method (6th edition) Bradford, England*, Bradford Dementia Research Group, Bradford University.

Kitwood, T. and Bredin, K. (1997) *Evaluating dementia care the DCM method (7th edition) Bradford, England*, Bradford Dementia Research Group, Bradford University.

Koenig, H.G., Meador, K.G., Cohen, H.J. and Blazer, D.G. (1988) Detection and treatment of major depression in older medically ill hospitalised patients, *International Journal of Psychiatric Medicine*, 160, 212–216.

Kraus, A.S., Spassoff, R.A., Beattie, E.J., Holden, D., Lawson, J.S., Rodeburg, J.M. and Woodcock, G.M. (1976) Elderly applicants to long-term institutions: their characteristics, health problems and state of mind, *Journal of the American Geriatric Society*, 24, 117–125.

Kutner, B., Fansel, D., Togo, A.M. and Langner, T.S. (1956) *Five Hundred over 60*, Russell Sage, New York.

Lacey, D. (1999) The evolution of care: a 100-year history of institutionalization of people with Alzheimer's Disease, *Journal of Gerontological Social Work*, 31, 3/4, 101–131.

Laing and Buisson (2001) *Care of Elderly People: Market Survey 2001*, Laing and Buisson, London.

Laing, W. (1998) *A Fair Price for Care? Disparities Between Market Rates for Nursing/ Residential Care and What State Funding Agencies Will Pay*, York Publishing Services, York.

Lawthom, R.L., Patterson, M. and West, M.A. (1996) *Measuring Organizational Climate*, (unpublished), Institute of Work Psychology, Sheffield.

Lawton, M.P. (1975) The Philadelphia Geriatric Center Morale Scale; a revision, *Journal of Gerontology*, 30, 85–89.

Lawton, M.P. (1983) Environment and other determinants of well-being in older people, *The Gerontologist*, 23, 349–57.

Lawton, M.P. (1991) A multidimensional view of quality of life in frail elders, in Birren, J.E., Lubben, J.E., Rowe, J.C. and Deutchman, D.E. (eds) *The Concept and Measurement of Quality of Life in the Frail Elderly*, Academic Press, San Diego.

Lazowski, D.A., Ecclestone, N.A., Myers, A.M., Paterson, D.H., Tudor-Locke, C., Fitzgerald, C., Jones, G., Shima, N. and Cunningham, D.A. (1999) A randomized outcome evaluation of group exercise programs in long-term care institutions, *Journals of Gerontology. Series A, Biological Sciences and Medical Sciences*, 54A, 12, M621-M628.

Lemke, S. and Moos, R.H. (1984) Coping with an intra-institutional relocation: behavioural change as a function of residents' personal resources, *Journal of Environmental Psychology*, 4, 137–151.

Levin, E., Moriarty, J. and Gorbach, P. (1994) *Better for the Break*, HMSO, London.

Lieberman, M.A. (1961) Relationship of mortality rates to entrance to a home for the aged, *Geriatrics*, 16, 515- 519.

Linn, M.W. (1966) A nursing home rating scale, *Geriatrics*, 21, 188–192.

Linn, M.W. (1977) Patient outcome as a measure of quality of nursing home care, *American Journal of Public Health*, 66, 337–344.

Lipsitz, L.A. (1994) The teaching nursing home: an educational and economic resource for geriatric training, *American Journal of Medicine*, 97, 4A, 245–265.

Locker, D. and Dunt, D. (1978) Theoretical and methodological issues in sociological studies of consumer satisfaction with medical care, *Social Science and Medicine*, 12, 283–292.

Lord, T.R. and Garner, J.E. (1993) Effect of music on Alzheimer patients, *Perceptual and Motor Skills*, 76, 2, 451–455.

Lunn, J., Chan, K., Donoghue, J., Riley, B. and Walley, T. (1997) A study of the appropriateness of prescribing in nursing homes, *The International Journal of Pharmacy Practice*, 5, 6–10.

Macdonald, J.D., Carpenter, G.I., Box, O., Roberts, A. and Sahu, S. (2002) Dementia and use of psychotropic medication in non 'Elderly Mentally Infirm' nursing homes in South East England, *Age and Ageing*, 31, 58–64.

Macfarlane, M. and Mugford M. (1984) *Birth Counts: Statistics of Pregnancy and Childbirth*, National Perinatal Epidemiology Unit in collaboration with OPCS, HMSO, London.

Maddox, G.L. and Douglas, E.B. (1973) Self assessment of health: a longitudinal study of elderly subjects, *Journal of Health and Social Behaviour*, 14, 87–93.

Mahoney, F. and Barthel, D. (1965) Functional evaluation: the Barthel Index, *Maryland State Medical Journal*, 14, 61–65.

Mangione, C.M., Marcantonio, E.R., Goldman, L., Cook, E.F., Donaldson, M.C., Sugarbaker, D.J., Poss, R. and Lee, T.H. (1993) Influence of age on measurement of health status in patients undergoing elective surgery, *Journal of The American Geriatrics Society*, 41, 377–385.

Manion, P.S. and Rantz, M. (1995) Relocation stress syndrome: A comprehensive plan for long term admission, *Geriatric Nursing*, 16, 3, 108–112.

Mann, A.H., Graham, N. and Ashby, D. (1984) Psychiatric illness in residential homes for the elderly: a survey in one London borough, *Age and Ageing*, 13, 257–265.

Mann, A.H., Schneider, J., Mozley, C., Levin, E., Blizard, R., Netten, A., Kharicha, K., Egelstaff, R., Abbey, A. and Todd, C. (2000) Depression and the response of residential homes to physical health need, *International Journal of Geriatric Psychiatry*, 15, 12, 1105–1112.

McCrea, D., Arnold, E., Marchevsky, D. and Kaufman, B.M. (1994) The prevalence of depression in medical outpatients, *Age and Ageing*, 23, 465–467.

McDowell, I. and Newell, C. (1996) *Measuring Health: A Guide to Rating Scales and Questionnaires*, Oxford U.P., New York.

McWilliam, C., Copeland, J.R.M., Dewey, M.E. and Wood, N. (1988) The Geriatric Mental State Examination as a case-study finding instrument in the community, *British Journal of Psychiatry*, 152, 205–208.

Mead, N., Bower, P. and Gask, L. (1997) Emotional problems in primary care: what is the potential for increasing the role of nurses? *Journal of Advanced Nursing*, 26, 5, 879–890.

Mikhail, M.L. (1992) Psychological responses to relocation to a nursing home, *Journal of Gerontological Nursing*, 18, 3, 35–39.

Mitchell, J. and Kemp, B.J. (2000) Quality of life in assisted living homes: a multidimensional analysis, *Journal of Gerontology: Psychological Sciences*, 55B, 2, P117-P127.

Moniz-Cook, E., Agar, S., Silver, M., Woods, R., Wang, M., Elston, C. and Win, T. (1998) Can staff training reduce behavioural problems in residential care for the elderly mentally ill?, *International Journal of Geriatric Psychiatry*, 13, 149–158.

Monk, D. (1985) *Social Grading on the National Readership Survey*, Joint Industry Committee of the National Readership Survey, London.

Moore, B.S., Newsome, J.A., Payne, P.L. and Tiansawad, S. (1993) Nursing research: quality of life and perceived health in the elderly, *Journal of Gerontological Nursing*, 19, 11, 7–14.

Moos, R.H. (1974) *Evaluating Treatment Environments: A Social Ecological Approach*, John Wiley and Sons, New York.

Moos, R.H. and Lemke, S. (1984) *Multiphasic Environmental Assessment Procedure (MEAP) Manual*, Social Ecology Laboratory, Stanford University, Palo Alto, California.

Moos, R.H. and Lemke, S. (1992) *Multiphasic Environmental Assessment Procedure Manuals: Multiphasic Environmental Assessment Procedure Users' Guide; Resident and Staff Information Form Manual; Sheltered Care Environment Scale Manual; Physical and Architectural Features Checklist Manual; Policy and Program Information Form Manual*, Center for Health Care Evaluation, Department of Veterans Affairs and Stanford University Medical Centers, Palo Alto, California.

Moos, R.H., Gauvain, M., Lemke, S., Max, W. and Mehren, B. (1979) Assessing the social environment of sheltered care settings, *The Gerontologist*, 19, 1, 74–82.

Mor, V. (2003) Benchmarking and quality in residential and nursing homes: lessons from the US, *International Journal of Geriatric Psychiatry*, 18, 3, 258–266.

Moriarty, J. and Webb, S. (2000) *Part of their Lives: Community Care for Older People with Dementia*, The Policy Press, Bristol.

Morris, J.N., Hawes, C., Fries, B.E., Phillips, C.D., Mor, V., Katz, S., Murphy, K., Drugovich, M.L. and Friedlob, A.S. (1990) Designing the National Resident Assessment Instrument for Nursing Homes, *The Gerontologist*, 30, 3, 293–307.

Moxon, S., Lyne, K., Sinclair, I., Young, P. and Kirk, C. (2001) Mental health in residential homes: a role for care staff, *Ageing and Society*, 21, 71–93.

Mozley, C.G., Huxley, P., Sutcliffe, C., Bagley, H., Burns, A., Challis, D. and Cordingley, L. (1999) 'Not knowing where I am doesn't mean I don't know what I like': cognitive impairment and quality of life responses in elderly people, *International Journal of Geriatric Psychiatry*, 14, 776–783.

Mozley, C.G., Challis, D., Sutcliffe, C., Bagley, H., Burns, A., Huxley, P. and Cordingley, L. (2000) Psychiatric symptomatology in elderly people admitted to nursing and residential homes, *Ageing and Mental Health*, 4, 2, 136–141.

Mozley, C., Schneider, J., Hart, C. and Duggan, S. (2003) Care Home Activity Project, *www.yorkhealthservices.org/viewpress.php3?id=44*.

Murphy, E. (1982) Social origins of depression in old age, *British Journal of Psychiatry*, 141, 135–142.

Murphy, E. (1983) Prognosis of depression in old age, *British Journal of Psychiatry*, 142, 111–119.

Murphy, E., Smith, R. and Lindsay, J. (1988) Increased mortality in late life depression, *British Journal of Psychiatry*, 152, 347–353.

Myers, F. and MacDonald, C. (1996) 'I was given options not choices': involving older users and carers in assessment and care planning, in Bland, R. (ed.) *Developing Services for Older People and their Families*, Jessica Kingsley, London.

Neal R.M. and Baldwin R.C. (1994) Screening for anxiety and depression in elderly medical outpatients, *Age and Ageing*, 23, 461–464.

Netten, A. (1993) *A Positive Environment? Physical and Social Influences on People with Senile Dementia in Residential Care*, Ashgate, Aldershot.

Netten, A., Darton, R., Bebbington, A., Forder, J., Brown, P. and Mummery, K. (2001a) Residential and nursing home care of elderly people with cognitive impairment: prevalence, mortality and costs, *Aging and Mental Health*, 5, 1, 14–22.

Netten, A., Darton, R., Bebbington, A. and Brown, P. (2001b) Residential or nursing home care? The appropriateness of placement decisions, *Ageing and Society*, 21, 3–23.

Netten, A., Darton, R. and Curtis L. (2001c) *Self-funded Admissions to Care Homes. A Report of Research Carried Out by the Personal Social Services Research Unit, University of Kent on behalf of the Department for Work and Pensions*, Department for Work and Pensions Research Report No. 159, Corporate Document Services, Leeds.

Netten, A., Darton, R. and Williams, J. (2002) The rate, causes and consequences of home closures, Discussion Paper 1741/2, Personal Social Services Research Unit, University of Kent at Canterbury.

Neugarten, B.L. (1974) Successful aging in 1970 and 1990, in Pfeiffer, E. (ed.) *Successful Aging: A Conference Report*, Center for the Study of Aging and Human Development, Durham, North Carolina.

Neugarten, B.L., Havighurst, R.J. and Tobin, S.S. (1961) The measurement of life satisfaction, *Journal of Gerontology*, 16, 134–143.

Newens, A.J., Forster, D.P. and Kay, D.W. (1993) Death certification after a diagnosis of presenile dementia, *Journal of Epidemiology and Community Health*, 47, 4, 293–297.

Norman, A. (1980) *Rights and Risks*, National Corporation for the Care of Older People, London.

North West Elderly Care Project (1994) Report commissioned by North West Association of Directors of Social Services, The Department of Health Social Services Inspectorate, Mersey Regional Health Authority, North West Regional Health Authority.

Novak, S., Johnson, J. and Greenwood, R. (1996) Barthel revisited: making guidelines work, *Clinical Rehabilitation*, 10, 128–134.

O'Connor, D.W., Pollitt, P.A., Treasure, F.P., Brook, C.P.B. and Reiss, B. (1989) The influence of education, social class and sex on Mini-Mental State Scores, *Psychological Medicine*, 19, 771–776.

O'Kell, S. (2002) *The Independent Care Homes Sector: Implications of Care Staff Shortages on Service Delivery*, York Publishing Services, York.

Office of National Statistics (2000) *Mortality Statistics: General Review of the Registrar General on Deaths in England and Wales, 2000*, HMSO, London.

Oleson, M., Heading, C., Shadick, K.M. and Bistodeau, J.A. (1994) Quality of life in long-stay institutions in England: nurse and resident perceptions, *Journal of Advanced Nursing*, 20, 23–32.

Oliver, J., Huxley, P., Bridges, K. and Mohamad, H. (1996) *Quality of Life and Mental Health Services*, Routledge, London.

Pahor, M., Guralnik, J.M., Chriscilles, E.A. and Wallace R.B. (1994) Use of laxative medication in older persons and associations with low serum albumin, *Journal of American Geriatric Society*, 42, 1, 50–56.

Parmalee, P.A., Katz, I.R. and Lawton, M.P. (1989) Depression among the institutionalised aged: assessment and prevalence estimation, *Journal of Gerontology*, 44, 1, 22–29.

Patrick, D.L. and Erickson, P. (1993) *Health Status and Health Policy: Quality of Life in Health Care Evaluation and Resource Allocation*, Oxford U.P., New York.

Patrick, D.L., Bush, J.W. and Chen, M.M. (1973) Methods for measuring levels of well-being for a health status index, *Health Services Research*, 8, 3, 228–245.

Paykel, E.S. (1991) Depression in women, *British Journal of Psychiatry*, 158, 22–29.

Payne, C. and a Group of North Tyneside Home Owners and Managers and Members of the Independent Inspection Team (1994) *Evaluating the Quality of Care: A Self Assessment Manual*, National Institute for Social Work, London.

Peace, S.M., Hall, J. and Hamblin, G.R. (1979) The quality of life of the elderly in residential care, Research Report No. 1, Survey Research Unit, The Polytechnic of North London.

Peace, S., Kellaher, L. and Willcocks, D. (1997) *Re-evaluating Residential Care*, Open University Press, Buckingham.

Pearce, D. and Britton, M. (1977) The decline in births: some socio-economic aspects, *Population Trends*, 7, 9–14.

Pearlman, R.A. and Uhlmann, R.F. (1988) Quality of life in chronic diseases: perceptions of elderly patients, *Journal of Gerontology*, 43, 2, 25–30.

Peet, S.M., Castleden, C.M., Potter, J.F. and Jagger, C. (1994) The outcome of a medical examination for applicants to Leicestershire homes for older people, *Age and Ageing*, 23, 65–68.

Phillips, C.D., Hawes, C., Mor, V., Fries, B.E. and Morris, J.N. (1996) *Evaluation of the Nursing Home Resident Assessment Instrument: Executive Summary*, Research Triangle Institute, North Carolina.

Phillips, C.D., Morris, J.N., Hawes, C., Fries, B.E., Mor, V., Nennstiel, M. and Iannacchione, V. (1997) Association of the Resident Assessment Instrument (RAI) with changes in function, cognition and psychosocial status, *Journal of the American Geriatric Society*, 45, 986–993.

Philp, I., Mutch, J. and Ogston, S. (1989) Can quality of life of old people in institutional care be measured?, *Journal of Clinical and Experimental Gerontology*, 11, 1 and 2, 11–19.

Philp, I., Mutch, W.J., Ballinger, B.R. and Boyd, L. (1991) A comparison of care in private nursing homes, geriatric and psychogeriatric hospitals, *International Journal of Geriatric Psychiatry*, 64, 253–258.

Pond, C.D., Mant, A., Bridges-Webb, C.M., Purcell, C., Eyland, E.A., Hewitt, H. and Saunders, N.A. (1990) Recognition of depression in the elderly: a comparison of the General Practitioner Opinions and the Geriatric Depression Scale, *Family Practice*, 7, 3, 190–194.

Primrose, W.R., Capewell, A.E., Simpson, G.K. and Smith, R.G. (1987) Prescribing patterns observed in registered nursing homes and long-stay geriatric wards, *Age and Ageing*, 16, 25–28.

Proctor, R., Stratton-Powell, H., Burns, A., Tarrier, N., Reeves, D., Emerson, E. and Hatton, C. (1998) An observational study to evaluate the impact of a specialist outreach team on the quality of care in nursing and residential homes, *Aging and Mental Health*, 2, 3, 232–238.

Quinn, M., Johnson, M., Andress, E., McGinnis, P. and Ramesh, M. (1999) Health characteristics of elderly personal care home residents, *Journal of Advanced Nursing*, 30, 2, 410–417.

Qureshi, K.N. and Hodkinson, H.M. (1974) Evaluation of a ten question mental test in the institutionalised elderly, *Age and Ageing*, 3, 152–157.

Qureshi, H. and Walker, A. (1989) *The Caring Relationship: Elderly People and Their Families*, Macmillan Education Ltd., Basingstoke.

Rafferty, J., Smith, R.G. and Williamson, J. (1987) Medical assessment of elderly persons prior to a move to residential care: a review of seven years experience in Edinburgh, *Age and Ageing*, 16, 10–12.

Rapp, S.R., Parisi, S.A., Walsh, D.A. and Wallace, C.E. (1988) Detecting depression in elderly medical inpatients, *Journal of Consulting and Clinical Psychology*, 56, 4, 509–513.

Raynes, N.V. (1995) *Standard Setting in Residential and Nursing Homes. Phase 1*, Report prepared for Manchester City Council Social Services Department, University of Huddersfield.

Raynes, N.V. (1996) *Standard Setting in Residential and Nursing Homes. Phase 2*, Report prepared for Manchester City Council Social Services Department, University of Huddersfield.

Raynes, N.V. (1998) Involving residents in quality specification, *Ageing and Society*, 18, 65–78.

Redfern, S.J. and Norman, I.J. (1990) Measuring the quality of nursing care: a consideration of different approaches, *Journal of Advanced Nursing*, 15, 1260–1271.

Reed, J. (1998) Gerontological nursing research — future directions, Paper given to the Agnet/Royal College of Nursing gerontological nursing research seminar, Regents College, London, December.

Reed, R. and Gilleard, C. (1995) Elderly patients' satisfaction with a community nursing service, in Wilson, G. (ed.) *Community Care: Asking the Users*, Chapman and Hall, London.

Reed, J. and Roskell-Payton, V. (1996) Constructing familiarity and managing the self: ways of adapting to life in nursing and residential homes for older people, *Ageing and Society*, 16, 543–560.

Reed, J., Roskell Payton, V. and Bond, S. (1998) The importance of place for older people moving into care homes, *Social Science and Medicine*, 46, 7, 859–867.

Richardson, J., Bedards, M. and Weaver, B. (2001) Changes in physical functioning in institutionalized older adults, *Disability and Rehabilitation*, 23, 15, 683–689.

Rizzo, J., House, R.J. and Lirtzman, S.J. (1970) Role conflict and ambiguity in complex organisations, *Administrative Science Quarterly*, 15, 150–163.

Robertson, M.C. (1996) What is old age?, *Public Health*, 110, 209–210.

Robinson, J.R. (1989) The natural history of mental disorder in old age — a long-term study, *British Journal of Psychiatry*, 154, 783–789.

Rosenberg, M. (1965) *Society and Adolescent Self-Image*, Princeton University Press, New Jersey.

Rosser, R. and Kind, P. (1978) A scale of valuations of states of illness; is there a social consensus?, *International Journal of Epidemiology*, 7, 347–358.

Roth, M. and Kay, D.W.K. (1956) Affective disorders arising in the senium, *Journal of Medical Science*, 102, 141–150.

Royal College of Nursing (1996) *Nursing Homes: Nursing Values*, Royal College of Nursing, London.

Royal College of Nursing (1997) *What a Difference a Nurse Makes: A report on the benefits of expert nursing to the clinical outcomes of older people in continuing care*, Royal College of Nursing, London.

Royal College of Physicians/British Geriatrics Society (1992) *High Quality Long Term Care for Elderly People: Guidelines and Audit Measures*, The Royal College of Physicians of London, London.

Royal Commission on Long Term Care (1999) *With Respect to Old Age: Long Term Care — Rights and Responsibilities, Community Care and Informal Care*, Cm 4192-II/3, The Stationery Office, London.

Ryan, A.A. and Scullion, H. (2000) Family and staff perceptions of the role of families in nursing homes, *Journal of Advanced Nursing*, 32, 3, 626–634.

Ryan, M.J., Wall, P.G., Adak, G.K., Evans, H.S. and Cowden, J.M. (1997) Outbreaks of infectious intestinal disease in residential institutions in England and Wales 1992–1994, *Journal of Infection*, 34, 1, 49–54.

Savartz, M.S. and Blazer, B.G. (1986) The distribution of effective disorders in old age, in Murphy, E. (ed.) *Affective Disorders in the Elderly*, Churchill Livingstone, Edinburgh.

Schneider, J., Mann, A.H., Levin, E., Netten, A., Mozley, C., Abbey, A., Egelstaff, R., Kharicha, K., Todd, C., Blizard, R. and Topan, C. (1997a) Quality of care: testing some measures in homes for elderly people, Discussion Paper 1245, Personal Social Services Research Unit, University of Kent at Canterbury.

Schneider, J., Mann A., Blizzard B. and Kharicha, K. (1997b) Quality of Residential Care for Elderly People: Phase II Study Extension, Discussion Paper 1304, Personal Social Services Research Unit, University of Kent at Canterbury.

Schneider, J., Mann, A.H. and Netten, A. (1997c) Residential care for elderly people: an exploratory study of quality measurement, *Mental Health Research Review*, 4, 2–15.

Schultz, R. and Brenner, G. (1977) Relocation of the aged: a review and theoretical analysis, *Journal of Gerontology*, 32, 323–333.

Shah, A. and De, T. (1998) Documented evidence of depression in medical and nursing case-notes and its implications in acutely ill geriatric inpatients, *International Psychogeriatrics*, 10, 2, June, 163–172.

Shah, I., Herbert, R., Lewis, S., Mahendran, R., Platt, J. and Bhattacharya, B. (1997) Screening for depression among acutely ill geriatric inpatients with a short geriatric depression scale, *Age and Ageing*, 26, 217–221.

Sharma, S.S., Aldous, J. and Robinson, M. (1994) Assessing applicants for Part III accommodation: is a formal clinical assessment worthwhile?, *Public Health*, 108, 91–97.

Shaw, S.M. and Opit, L.J. (1976) The need for supervision in the elderly receiving long term prescribed medication, *British Medical Journal*, 1, 28, 505–507.

Sheikh, J.I. and Yesavage, J.A. (1986) Geriatric Depression Scale (GDS). Recent evidence and development of a shorter form, *Clinical Gerontology*, 5, 165–173.

Shepherd, G., Muijen, M., Dean, R. and Cooney, M. (1996) Residential care in hospital and in the community — quality of care and quality of life, *British Journal of Psychiatry*, 168, 448–456.

Shergill, S.S., Shankar, K.K., Seneviratna, K. and Orrell, M.W. (1999) The validity and reliability of the Health of the Nation Outcome Scales (HoNOS) in the elderly, *Journal of Mental Health*, 8, 5, 511–521.

Sikorska-Simmons, E. (2001) Development of an instrument to measure resident satisfaction with assisted living, *Journal of Applied Gerontology*, 20, 1, 57–73.

Sinclair, I. (1990) Residential care: the research reviewed, in Sinclair, I., Parker, R., Leat, D. and Williams, J. (eds) *The Kaleidoscope of Care*, National Institute for Social Work, London.

Slevin, M.L., Plant, H., Lynch, D., Drinkwater, J. and Gregory, W.M. (1988) Who should measure quality of life, the doctor or the patient?, *British Journal of Cancer*, 57, 109–112.

Sloane, P.D., Zimmerman, S., Brown, L.C., Ives, T.J. and Walsh, J.F (2002) Inappropriate medication prescribing in residential care/assisted living facilities, *Journal of the American Geriatrics Society*, 50, 6, 1001–1011.

Snedecor, G. and Cochran, W. (1980) *Statistical Methods (7th edition)*, Iowa State University Press, Iowa.

Spector, W. D. and Takada, H. A. (1999) Characteristics of nursing homes that affect resident outcomes, *Journal of Aging and Health*, 3, 427-54.

Spitzer, W.O., Dobson, A.J., Hall, J., Chesterman, E., Levi, J., Shepherd, R., Battista, R.N. and Catchlove, B.R. (1981) Measuring the quality of life of cancer patients, *Journal of Chronic Diseases*, 34, 585–597.

Steiner, A. (2001) Intermediate care — a good thing?, *Age and Ageing*, 30, S3, 33–39.

Stewart, K., Challis, D., Carpenter, I. and Dickinson, E. (1999) Assessment approaches for older people receiving social care: content and coverage, *International Journal of Geriatric Psychiatry*, 14, 147–156.

Stott, D.J., Dutton, M., Williams, B.O. and Macdonald, J. (1990) Functional capacity and mental status of elderly people in long term care in West Glasgow, *Health Bulletin*, 48, 17–24.

Stuck, A.E., Zwahlen, H.G., Neuenschwander, B.E., Meyer Schweizer, R.A., Bauen, G. and Beck, J.C. (1995) Methodologic challenges of randomised controlled studies on in-home comprehensive geriatric assessment: the Eiger Project: evaluation of in-home geriatric health visits in elderly residents, *Aging: Clinical and Experimental Research*, 7, 3, 218–223.

Sutcliffe, C., Cordingley, L., Burns, A., Godlove Mozley, C., Bagley, H., Huxley, P. and Challis, D. (2000) A new version of the Geriatric Depression Scale for nursing and residential home populations: the Geriatric Depression Scale (Residential) (GDS-12R), *International Psychogeriatrics*, 12, 2, 173–181.

Szalai, A. (1980) The meaning of comparative research on the quality of life, in Szalai, A. and Andrews, F.M. (eds) *The Quality of Life*, Sage, London.

Taylor, J.C. and Bowers, D.G. (1972) *Survey of Organisations: a Machine Read Standardised Questionnaire Instrument*, Institute of Social Research, University of Michigan, Ann Arbor.

Taylor, M. (ed.) with Brice, J., Buck, N. and Prentice, E. (1995) *British Household Panel Survey User Manual*, University of Essex, Colchester.

Thomas, P., Garry, P. and Goodwin, J. (1986) Morbidity and mortality in an initially healthy elderly sample: findings after five years of follow-up, *Age and Ageing*, 15, 105–110.

Thomas, W. (1994) *The Eden Alternative: Nature, Hope and Nursing Homes*, Eden Alternative Foundation, New York.

Thomas, W. (1996) *Life Worth Living*, Vanderwyk and Burnham, Massachussetts.

Timko, C. and Moos, R.H. (1991a) Assessing the quality of residential programs: methods and applications, *Adult Residential Care Journal*, 5, 113–129.

Timko, C. and Moos, R.H. (1991b) A typology of social climates in group residential facilities for older people, *Journal of Gerontology: Social Sciences*, 46, 3, S160-S169.

Tobin, S.S. and Lieberman, M.M. (1976) *Last Home for the Aged*, Jossey-Bass, San Francisco, California.

Tombaugh, T.N. and McIntyre, N.J. (1992) The Mini-Mental State Examination: a comprehensive review, *Journal of The American Geriatric Society*, 40, 922–935.

Townsend, P. (1957) *The Family Life of Old People: An Enquiry in East London*, Routledge and Kegan Paul, London.

Townsend, P. (1962) *The Last Refuge*, Routledge and Kegan Paul, London.

Tuke, S. (1813) *Description of The Retreat*, Process Press, York (reprinted 1996), edited by Professor Kathleen Jones.

Tulle-Winton, E. (1995) Do you remember your social worker? Identification and recall problems in user surveys, in Wilson, G. (ed.) *Community Care: Asking the Users*, Chapman and Hall, London.

Tune, P. and Bowie, P. (2000) The quality of residential and nursing-home care for people with dementia, *Age and Ageing*, 29, 325–328.

Tunstall, J. (1966) *Old and Alone: A Sociological Study of Old People*, Routledge and Kegan Paul, London.

Turnham, H. (2001) *OBRA '87 Summary*, National Long Term Care Ombudsman Resource Center, *http://www.ltcombudsman.org/ombpublic/ 49_346_1023.cfm*.

Ulfarsson, J. and Robinson, B.E. (1994) Preventing falls and fractures, *Journal of the Florida Medical Association*, 81, 11, 763–767.

Van Dijk, P.T., Dippel, D.W., Van Der Meulen, J.H. and Habbema, J.D., (1996) Co-morbidity and its effect on mortality in nursing home patients with dementia, *Journal of Nervous and Mental Disorders*, 184, 3, 180–187.

Vardon, V.M. and Blessed, G. (1986) Confusion ratings and Abbreviated Mental Test performance: a comparison, *Age and Ageing*, 15, 139–144.

Wade, D. (1992) *Measurement in Neurological Rehabilitation*, Oxford University Press, Oxford.

Wade, D.T. and Collin, C. (1988) The Barthel ADL Index: a standard measure of physical disability?, *International Disability Studies*, 10, 64–67.

Wade, S. and Skinner, A. (2001) Student placements in nursing homes, *Nursing Older People*, 13, 2, 14–17.

Wagner, G. (1988) *Residential Care: A Positive Choice. Report of the Independent Review of Residential Care*, HMSO, London.

Wall, T.D., Bolden, R.J., Borrill, C.S., Carter, A.J., Golya, D.A., Hardy, G.E., Haynes, C.E., Rick, J.E., Shapiro, D.A. and West, M.A. (1997) Minor psychiatric disorder in NHS trust staff: occupational and gender differences, *British Journal of Psychiatry*, 171, 519–523.

Warr, P., Cook, J. and Wall, T. (1979) Scales for the measurement of some work attitudes and aspects of psychological well-being, *Journal of Occupational Psychology*, 52, 129–148.

Warr, P.B. (1990) The measurement of wellbeing and other aspects of mental health, *Journal of Occupational Psychology*, 63, 193–210.

Wells, Y.D. and Jorm, A.E. (1987) Evaluation of a special nursing home unit for dementia sufferers, *Australian and New Zealand Journal of Psychiatry*, 21, 524–531.

West, M.A. and Savage, Y. (1988) Coping with stress in health visiting, *Health Visitor*, 61, 366–368.

Wild, K.V. and Kaye, J.A. (1998) The rate of progression of Alzheimer's disease in the later stages: evidence from the Severe Impairment Battery, *Journal of the International Neuropsychological Society*, 4, 5, 512–516.

Wilkin, D. and Hughes, B. (1987) Residential care of elderly people: the consumers' views, *Ageing and Society*, 7, 2, 175–202.

Wilkin, D. and Thompson, C. (1989) *Users' Guide to Dependency Measures for Elderly People*, Social Services Monograph, University of Sheffield.

Willcocks, D., Peace, S. and Kellaher, L. (1987) *Private Lives in Public Places*, Tavistock, London.

Wing, J., Beevor, A., Park, S., Hadden, S. and Burns, A. (1998) Health of the Nation Outcome Scales (HoNOS), *British Journal of Psychiatry*, 172, 11–18.

Wolfensberger, W. (1972) *The Principle of Normalization in Human Services*, National Institute on Mental Retardation, Toronto.

Wolfensberger, W. and Glenn, L. (1978) *PASS3, Program Analysis of Service Systems: a method for the quantitative evaluation of human services: Field Manual*, National Institute on Mental Retardation, York University, Toronto.

Yawney, B. and Slover, D.I. (1973) Relocation of the elderly, *Social Work*, 18, May, 86–93.

Yesavage, J.A. (1988) Geriatric Depression Scale, *Psychopharmacological Bulletin*, 24, 709–710.

Yesavage, J.A., Brink, T.L., Rose, T.L., Lum, O., Huang, V., Day, M. and Leirer, V.O. (1983) Development and validation of a Geriatric Depression Screening Scale, *Journal of Psychiatric Research*, 17, 37–49.

Youll, P.J. and McCourt-Perring, C. (1993) *Raising Voices: Ensuring Quality in Residential Care*, HMSO, London.

Zimmerman, D., Karon, S., Arling, G., Clarke, B.R., Collins, E., Ross, R. and Sainfort, F. (1995) The development and testing of Nursing Home Quality Indicators, *Health Care Financing Review*, 16, 107–27.

Name Index

257

Subject Index